Fitness Business 101

What The Certifications Don't Teach You

Steve Washuta

CONTENTS

ACKNOWLEDGMENTS

To all who helped me along my journey. Paying it forward.

1 - INTRODUCTION/ABOUT ME

"The only life worth living is dedicated in substantial part to good outcomes one cannot possibly survive to see." – **Charlie Munger, <u>Poor Charlie's Almanack</u>**

I distinctly remember walking into the office on a cold January morning in New York City knowing that it was going to be my last day at work. I was sitting in midtown Manhattan, 40 floors up, looking out over Times Square wondering how I got there, and how I felt I was as far away from what I wanted to be doing in life, as was the sidewalk below me. Those of us who chose the route of corporate hacks only to feel as if you've made a wrong turn somewhere understand one another. This may be why you are reading this right now. Maybe you've been doing yoga for the past five years and enjoy teaching your family members positions, or you're the go-to person in your crew when discussing the best leg exercises. You may also be fresh out of school with a lifelong passion in health, or as a long-time Fitness Industry Teacher (FIT). You may also be career transitioning as you recently noticed your skill set in the health/fitness industry is or could be unique. Whatever the reason, now that you've realized your passion, I can show you the route to monetize it while doing what it is we are best at as FIT — helping others.

I played football, baseball, and basketball from the age of 6 religiously all year round. If I wasn't playing a sport, I was working in the off-season training for it. I was unknowingly building my fitness business long before I could drive a car. I learned drills, lifting techniques, kinesiology, stretching routines, nutrition, recovery, all while simply having fun. When I went off to college I majored in Public Relations. PR is (I'll never forget the definition) creating and maintaining relations between an organization and its constituents through strategic two-way communication. I loved the idea of being the representative of an organization and being able to honestly and openly build relations with the goal of always selecting the best courses of action.

Upon graduating, I joined a PR firm in Manhattan. It was located in Chelsea, a stone's throw to Madison Square Garden, and had a great mix of trendy and touristy. I loved my coworkers, the clients, but absolutely hated the work and daily grind. I then moved on to a hedge fund for two years and felt the same emptiness. Every day there seemed to be someone getting fired, and my level of importance in the company assured me it was only a matter of time. I was hopping on four different trains and subways for a 90-minute commute only to sit down all day answering emails at such a rapid pace that my mouse hand pointer finger was becoming arthritic. I eventually asked myself why waste my time answering emails for other people to mark off their to-do list, while neglecting to do mine. Actual work was rarely getting done, and I wasn't fulfilled. Well, now that I wasting five years of school and 100k in loans, I guess I don't have many other options except to stick with it, right? Wrong. Fortunately, I understood my happiness was of the utmost importance long term. You do too because you're still reading this.

We have the tendency to look at major life decisions as proverbial roads or paths. If you choose the left path rather than the right path, there is some butterfly effect that propels you into another realm of existence in which you're forever stuck. I implore you to think of your career path differently. Imagine that instead of a linear path, you have a horizontal line with an infinite number of careers, and for the sake of visual context each career is represented by a mason jar sitting on that line. Each jar holds a specific number of marbles until it is filled, and when it is, you've earned an expertise in that profession. Every marble represents a characteristic, situation, skill, or thought you have about a particular career. If I personally were to look at all my mason jars, I may have only a few marbles in the "Artist" jar. However, from my past experiences with sports, exercise, and passion for nutrition and health, I may have my "Personal Trainer & Health Coach" jar half-filled just from life experiences prior to making the leap. What scares most of us is the thought of starting over, but you now know that your mason jar was being filled all along the way and is waiting for you to drop in more marbles.

It's a daunting task to jump into a new career, or to even slightly shake up what we are currently doing and switch business models. When I changed careers, I moved across the country, spent all of my savings, and was sleeping on a friend's couch. I was lost. I dropped off my laughable resume to every gym in my new town, and only received one call. That call was the catalyst to my entire career in the industry because I learned how <u>not</u> to run a business.

At 34 years old, I have had over 25,000 personal training sessions, and a long waiting list of clientele. I have never felt richer or more refreshed than I do today. Forget financially, I am speaking purely from the freedom of never thinking about money. I wake up every day excited to work with people I consider friends, all while helping them reach their goals. I don't wait for the weekend, I don't check my bank account daily, and I don't dream of fantasy vacations. I made my life the vacation.

There are rarely times in life where all the stop lights are green. If you're waiting for "the right time" to change careers or fix your current business model, chances are you will take it to the grave. What you need to do is limit the risk factors when making big decisions. I am here to help you do just that.

The co-founder of the Princeton Review, Adam Robinson, once said, "People who have found happiness, love and long-term financial success all have one thing in common, they achieved it doing them indirectly." As a FIT, your priorities and attention shouldn't be focused on immediate success through marketing strategies, or building the best Instagram page, or even solely on your finances, but rather on doing the right things, little by little, day by day, in the space you work and live in. The tasks that involve your daily training sessions, coupled with your own personal development and your clients' goals are what will matter. If I could only emphasize one point from this book it would be to wake up every day with unrelenting focus and desire to help your clients in any fashion necessary, because the rest is easy and will fall right into place.

Becoming the ultimate FIT depends on your willingness to become a great listener, create positivity out of all situations, and realize your skill sets.

Throughout this book I'm going to jump back and forth; I'll have what I call "zoom in" for techniques, strategies, business details, and "zoom out" for philosophical and psychological tips and motivation. Learning both right and left side brain techniques is a must for success in this industry. Not everything can be boiled down into a formula. We have emotions and intuitive logic that come into play when building connections with our prospective clients for life. I'll teach you ways to use your skill sets and natural coaching abilities to compound your business as a FIT.

"What if I don't have any skills or know exactly what my skill set is?" We all have skill sets that don't jump out at us instantly no matter how many times they've been beaten into our skull. Take some time to think about family, friends, coworkers, teachers, and even superior's compliments toward you throughout your life.

While on vacation in Atlantic City, NJ, in my early 20's, I was waiting in line for the men's room. A man in his late 70's and I struck up a conversation about nothing and everything. "You're going to make it in this world, you're a great listener", he told me by the time we left the bathroom. I assumed this man was drunk, as we barely had six minutes of conversation. In hindsight, hundreds of people have paid me similar compliments in my life, and I let the compliments roll off my back. REALIZE YOUR SKILL SET. Mine was working one-on-one with people. What comes easy for you? What is it that your friends and family consistently tell you that you're great at? FIT need to marry their fitness skills and knowledge to their God-given or developed skills and let the duo shine. For some it's specifically social, cognitive, emotional, memory, or physiological, while most of us are a hybrid of one or more of these.

Whatever your path was to get you to this point, you've developed a host of other skill sets that can and will fuse with your niche in the fitness industry. Your mason jar has filled up more than you can imagine. We will delve deeper into finding what your niche is, or should be, and where your skill sets lie.

For now, the hard part is over. You've discovered that helping people in the realm of health and fitness is your passion. Now it's time to realize and develop your strengths in the fitness and health industry, and never stop chasing your dream. There are endless ways to monetize it, and I'm here to help you expedite your fitness business journey; but understand this: caring for your clients, and truly feeling passionately about helping them arrive at their goals is the only tool I can guarantee leads you to success. If that isn't something you currently have, or something that can't be awakened inside of you, there are no techniques, marketing strategies, or tools that will bring you success as a FIT.

2 - SCARY QUESTIONS

"Success is best achieved by minimizing losses and not taking large risks." –
Unknown

**I don't have any experience or certifications, so how do I compete
with others and where do I start?**

You've already started. The fact that you are here puts you years ahead of
anyone else who is trying to go down the same path. There are sand traps in
this industry that I have watched others get caught in or have gotten caught
in myself. Most people in this industry are stuck. I am here to make sure
you will avoid these by being efficient and effective. We will get to your
education and/or certifications after this, but first it's best to mentally map
out what an ideal day would be like for you. Write a few lines down or say it
out loud. The following are examples:

-Teaching yoga on the beach to 50 people at 7:30 a.m. and again at 6:00
   p.m. making $1,000 a day…cash.
-Personal training in my in-home fitness facility working exclusively
   with 10 clients who pay me $500/each month to meet with me
   twice a week in helping them improve speed and strength.
-Running a sport-specific clinic on the weekends for all ages charging
   $50/per person and having over 100 attendees per day.
-Teaching an outdoor bootcamp class at noon to local retirees or stay-
   at-home moms four days a week with a $20/per class charge and a
   weekly attendance of over 200.
-Hosting weekly nutritional/wellness talks via webcam to hundreds of
   subscribers paying monthly fees.

Did you have anything similar in mind? If so, I've done all of this, and it was actually ridiculously easy once I learned the few key strategies to running a fitness/health business. Now you can skip the first few years of painstaking trial and error, cancelations, low turnout numbers, and small pay checks. I'm excited to show you how simple it really is, as long as the passion and vision you have are coupled with my strategies.

How can I shift careers, and expect to not take a pay cut?

My financials year to year from training looked something like this: Year 1 – 15k, Year 2 – 20k, Year 3 – 25k. It took me four years before I made it over 30k, five years before I made it over 50k, and seven years before I made 100k. It wasn't because I was "earning it the hard way", or that it was just part of the growth process, or that I didn't have a good enough certification or skill set…it was because I had zero guidance on how to actually run a fitness business! Certifications give you little to no insight whatsoever on how to gain clientele, work with people, and earn money. I want to make sure you do not have to go through that arduous process of cancellations and low clientele, and I want you to have the confidence and tools to fill your schedule.

Ok, but really, what certifications/education do I need?

You'll get 10 different answers from 10 different people on this question. I want to be clear and emphasize this: Certifications/Education gets your foot in the door, but they do not represent your actual skill set.

I have trained alongside people with who have their Masters in Exercise Physiology and held a dozen top level certifications costing more than 5k collectively, who had trouble booking 10 sessions a week. I have worked with yoga instructors coming off of two years of specialized training who couldn't fill a class of eight. I have worked with registered dieticians who averaged one appointment a day because they could not connect with people on a psychological level. You are stepping into an industry where people trust you with their bodies, and subsequently with their mental health. Learning ways (which will be discussed in the upcoming chapters) and enjoying the process of building connections will be of much more value than endless certifications, most of which the paying clients won't even be familiar with anyway.

If your plan is to work as your own boss in your home or elsewhere, you may not need any specific certification. If you decide to work for someone, the business typically requires you have one. Which one? That depends on the specific business. The nutritional counseling world is its own beast and very different then fitness. States have their own specific rules and regulations from getting paid to giving out nutritional advice. The fitness world, however, is an unregulated and decentralized market. Meaning, you could actually have no qualifications or certifications and still work with people in fitness. For the sake of professionalism, most fitness businesses have their own set requirements for the certifications they trust. How do they decide that? Do you own an iPhone or Android? After you answer that, you probably inferred that I was going to judge you on your choice. Why? Because people are tribal by nature and we instinctually pick teams. Typically, the certification held by the highest-level employee is the most respected for that specific business. If I am a director of a fitness facility and I hold an American Council on Exercise (ACE) certification for Group Fitness, I know what ACE teaches, I understand their concepts, and I trust them. Therefore, I am more likely to hire someone with the same certification. That is why it is important to dig into the business website of your preferred studio/facility or call them to find out what certifications their managers or top-level instructors hold.

For those of you who are aiming to be personal trainers, I have a detailed list of the top certifications and rankings in various categories that can be found on my blog: www.stevewashuta.com/swellness.

However, before you go there, your first step should be a few google searches of people in particular you feel have a skill set similar to yours, or ones you wish to model your skill set after. Once you find them, write down those certifications(s). My link above accomplishes the remainder of the research you need to do as I rank the various certs in these categories: Price – Prestige – Difficulty. The price will give you an idea of the cost and annual fees, the prestige will give insight into the industry's views on that particular certification, and the difficulty will rank the difficulty in attaining the certification (tests, education, etc.).

Should I start my own fitness business or work for someone first?

Like anything else in life, there are pros and cons to both sides. Starting your own business for many initially seems to be fiscally daunting. You'll have to have the capital for equipment, space, marketing, etc. However, long term you won't have to pay a percentage of your profits to whomever you work underneath. There is no one right way, but there are a lot of wrong ways. Below is a list of questions that after answering will guide you to the proper path suited for you at this time.

- If given any equipment and space you desire, would you feel confident enough to run a class/session/training/teaching tomorrow?
- Have you lived in your city/community for more than 2 years?
- Do you currently partake weekly in the fitness medium you are trying to teach? (i.e., I want to be a yoga instructor; do you take yoga classes regularly?).
- Do you have a social media presence?
- Do you have a job or leisure activity which puts you in daily contact with the local community?

If you answered YES to the majority of these, you most likely COULD jump right into owning your own fitness business. However, I always recommend to first at least working part-time for someone. This gives you a chance to network and be around people who already love to do what you teach. It also allows you to learn from other instructors and develop your niche (which we will expand on later).

If you said NO to majority of these, you will be much better off starting to work for a business/person who is already established. This will give you time to hone your craft, gain credibility in your community, build a stronger sense of self confidence, and be focused on networking/learning rather than being burdened by your personal fitness financial investment. It is easier than you think to land a job, and I will go over an almost foolproof plan to getting your foot in the door in the next chapters.

I don't think I know enough (exercises, information, routines) but I enjoy working with people. How can I get all the tools?

This is the easiest part. There is never a need to reinvent the wheel in fitness/health. However, you won't learn everything by simply reading books or getting certified. You will learn the basics through attending sessions or classes, certifications, shadowing, reading, and researching. Later in the book, I will go over the "Central 7", the seven bedrock movements of fitness. Once you understand the basics and the Central 7, you can use a handful of variables interchangeably to have an endless bag of tricks. Let's go ahead and get specific. For one exercise (push-ups), I can give you 10 different ways to do it without blinking and eye: 3-second eccentric (controlling it on the way down), 3-second concentric (controlling it on the way up), half pushups, feet on an unstable surface (ball), hands on an unstable surface (bosu), diamond push-ups, wide arm push-ups, push-up to clap, push-up to knee ups, push-up to pike toe-touch.

This isn't simply because of my knowledge in personal training. It's about understanding a few key variables and interchanging them giving you exponential options for exercises when combined with fitness toys.

If you are a coach/counselor (health, sport specific coach, etc.), it's exactly the same. There is no need to reinvent the wheel. It's about changing up key variables like timing, positioning, items (food, exercises, routines, etc.), and difficulty — using the bedrock movements or principles in your given health and fitness realm to give you endless option of tricks and tools.

Am I wrong for feeling like I do not have the time or money to just change careers?

Yes, you are. Very wrong in fact, but it's normal. I felt the same way and was scared out of my mind during the whole process. I can break this down in multiple ways. First, you are here because you deserve better. Forget about the fact you will be making more money in a short period of time, but if you don't currently love what you are doing, do you want to still be there in 10 years? Who is to say your current employer couldn't just let you go tomorrow? Tim Ferris describes an excellent fear exercise in his book, *The 4-Hour Work Week*. You imagine and then write out the worst possible scenario before you make a job-related decision. I recommend this. For me, the worst possible scenario if I quit my job and moved across the country at 26 was that in 6 months' time I would have still been unhappy and found my way back home, exactly where I left off. Wait, exactly where I left off?

YES. Why wouldn't I take that risk then? Give it a shot and write out your worst fears about starting or changing your current model of being a FIT. Moonlighting and learning/working part time is always an option. At worst, finding your way after reading this book will allow you to have a back-up plan if you don't decide to jump in with two feet. At best, you can transition into your ideal day-to-day life doing what it is you love and making more money then you did in your previous rat race job.

Secondly, this isn't just a "career change", it's a long-term investment. 80 billion US dollars! Read that number again. 80 billion US dollars was put into the health/wellness industry by consumers in 2017. That number does not include the billions spent on surgeries that require rehab and subsequently working to get stronger with FIT. This number is only going up. From 4-year-old children taking golf lessons, to 84-year-old seniors in Parkinson's Boxing classes, people are paying money for lessons, teaching, coaching, and other experts in our industry. Look at your Instagram, Facebook, billboards, etc., and you'll see that fitness and health ads are everywhere in the teen, young adult, and mid adult age ranges. Not to mention the growth curve is on the verge of shooting up exponentially now more than ever due to the baby boomers. By 2030, more than 20% of the US population will be over 65. That means right now, in the next 12 years, 20% of the population is trying to stay young and fit going into retirement! This is our key. That is the age range that has the most expendable income to work with you (or to pay for their family members to work with you). The majority of my clients are in this age range, and I will go over targeting that clientele specifically later in the book.

How does the pay structure work?

Typically, the dollar amount itself is geographic-specific. A yoga class or a 5-pack of personal training sessions in Los Angeles, CA is double of what it is in Savannah, GA. However, it's all relative as the cost of living is much higher in Los Angeles. Structurally however, let's go over standard pay formats for FIT:

> **Own your Business:** You can work from your home or from a facility you own, outdoors, or rent time/space from a facility. Many trainers prefer to pay a fixed monthly payment, like renting from a facility, having no boss, and doing their own marketing. They can

then charge whatever price they feel appropriate and keep all of the profits. When facilities allow you to work in their space while you run your own business, it typically is a great option. You do, however, have to account for your own taxes, but you will also get to write off many of the purchases.

Percentage-Based Commissions: You will find most facilities structure payment this way and will put you as an independent contractor. You can be hired on full time (benefits) and still make commission, but that is rare in this industry (always look for that, however). Most FIT are commissioned on how many sessions/classes/clients are worked with throughout a given time period. You can also work as a commission-based employee part time. Percentages range anywhere from 35%-80% (but typically closer to 60%) depending on location, experience, skill level, facility type, and negotiation power. Negotiation power is important, and I will go over that later in the book.

Salary: Some FITs are salaried. You train people as part of the salary or make a very small percentage commission on top of your salary. This normally entails desk duties or other tasks outside of standard teaching.

I want to be a fitness professional on a part-time basis only. Does this all apply for me too?

Of course. Every piece of information I will give you or have given you thus far can be used for part time as well. It will be more difficult from a time management perspective, but if you aren't in any rush, you can still implement all the techniques and strategies from both the zoom in and zoom out perspectives. The goal should eventually be only working part time hours and making full time money. I will go over that in the marketing strategies.

I want to build my business online (through Instagram, Facebook, Website, Twitter, etc.). Can I do it?

Sure. Thousands of people make great money in the fitness industry while never being face to face with clients, or even leaving their own homes.

However, it's difficult, time consuming, and the tactics to build your business this way are risky. Online fitness is the single most competitive sub-market in the industry. It costs almost nothing to set up a camera or blog, and no certifications are needed, so they pop up in droves. Most of the people making videos and claiming to be coaches or experts on social media sites are not making any real money. I have a friend who has 14k Instagram followers and has been writing online blogs for years. He'll never make half of what I pull in, and ultimately he puts more work into marketing on a day-to-day basis than I ever have to. Instagram doesn't provide value, it provides pictures. Building your social media (Chapter 4) is important, and I will go over key tactics, but it's typically a mistake to focus on that when you're starting. Your work should drive people to your social media rather than your social media drive people to work with you. It is only done the other way in rare circumstances. Build your trust and authority and then transfer it to the social media aspects. If you feel you already have a large following and name recognition in your social media circles concerning your expertise, you can certainly make it your nice/sub-niche and be a FIT through that medium. But understand that it can be difficult to show authority when you haven't had actual real-world experience. If your time and energy is spent online trying to convey to people that you are an expert, you're forgoing the actual opportunity of learning skills to become that expert you desire to be. We will talk more about social media marketing, videos, etc. in the later chapters.

If I start tomorrow, how long before I begin making money?

Honestly, if you're driven, you could make money tomorrow. However, it's not about short-term profits. It's about building your reputation, skill set, and coupling that with a few key marketing and business strategies. You benefit most from zeroing in on people who want to work with you, and whom you want to work with. This way, you'll have less client turnover, be recommended at a furious rate, and be gaining clientele faster than you can manage. If you start working with people before you are ready, or work with the wrong people, you will rob yourself of a constant/consistent revenue stream. Your goal is to maintain a handful of loyal followers for life, not to keep chasing down one and done sessions. There is a difference between motion and progress. You are only going to take the steps that help you move forward and let your business build itself passively. You want people to be spreading the word about your skill-set while you're working — it's free marketing! If your focus is on finding the next person rather than truly honing your craft and being the best FIT, you'll always be chasing down business rather than letting business come to you. The strategies given throughout the next chapters will shed light on how exactly to do this. I promise if you follow the path, you'll enjoy the process and the money will come before you even realize you're finished.

I'm currently working as a FIT, but there are only so many hours in the day and I'm not making enough money…what can I do?

This entire book will be filled with ways you can help make more money and become the best version of a FIT. However, from a financial standpoint I'll point out a few quick tips:

If you work for yourself, you have some options:

Charge More! Your time is of the utmost value as it's limited. Even if you have clients who refuse to pay more, you will fill that time with people who are eventually willing to do so. You are worth whatever you believe you are worth. You can always bring the prices down if you feel things are not going well, but do not shy away from high-priced hours as long as you are providing what you and your client believe is a truly high value experience.

You may need to start hiring people and taking a percentage. After reading the book and understanding the strategies to gain clientele, you can offload them to people who work for you. This will allow you to make money passively and allowing your business to truly flourish. You need to gain the trust of your clients before you offload them to others, and you'll have to make sure you use techniques taught here when training your future employees so that they keep a consistent structured business model that mirrors yours. Remember three key factors when going about this process: Create organizational hierarchy, develop a detailed position description, and personally train the employee properly.

If you work for someone:

Negotiate. If you are working for a company, you are way more valuable to them than they are to you. Chances are for every dollar they are paying you, you are making them two dollars. On top of taking a large percentage of what you make during each hour you work with someone, they are also benefiting from your connections and professionalism in keeping people happy, which in turn leads to them paying for other costs (memberships, packages, food etc.). That means you are essentially costing them nothing yet keeping their doors open. Review average percentages in your area, present your credentials, and negotiate what you believe is fair. Also, use the connections you have made inside your company. The people you work with are friendly and familiar with you and will become your greatest allies. They can aid in your negotiation if they know they are likely to lose you due to the company's stubbornness to not give you a raise. Losing an employee and having to retrain and reestablish personal connections with members is much more difficult for the company in our industry than in a standard pencil pusher job where you don't have as much person to person contact. In the later chapters, I will hit on how to gain leverage and the art of negotiation.

3 - FINDING YOUR NICHE

"You don't need to be the best at one thing, to be uniquely qualified to do something" – **Sam Harris**

Walking into my first day on the job as a FIT, I was repeatedly asked one question more than any other, "What's your specialty?" At that point, I had a background in nutrition (although not a registered nutritionist/dietician) so I simply said, "I don't know". I went from a motivated rookie to a lost soul in a matter of one day. I was angry with myself; "What the hell, Steve, you don't have a specialty?!" I decided to stress that nutrition was my passion, and yet took on a few different fitness training tools to separate myself. I became certified and then taught myself every movement imaginable (using the Central 7 method which we will discuss later) for the TRX suspension trainer which at the time was just becoming a mainstream fitness tool. I then gladly took part in learning the Pilates reformer and the accompanying techniques as it was a female-dominated industry, and gender leverage would be to my advantage. Both of these tools helped pave the way for my career. It wasn't about what I selected specifically, but why. I want to show you the "why", and help you conquer becoming an "expert" in a specific health and fitness genre, while still garnering respect as a qualified professional in your general field.

In order to separate yourself from the crowd and develop into an authority as a FIT, you are going to have to find your niche. You may already have one or have thought about how you can separate yourself. Many times, its past circumstances and passion that guides you toward your niche, like working with children as a tennis instructor because of fond memories you had as a child with your coach. Other situations dictate the particular niche due to its need like not having any female Olympic weight lifting coaches at your fitness facility. Regardless, I have put together a foolproof way to ensure you are choosing the correct path. *Shadowing* will help you understand the industry and give you a sense of what niche you should connect with. Coupled with *Shadowing*, understanding your *FIT Style and Specialty* will give insight into what type of teacher you are, and the avenues best served to lead you toward your niche.

Now that we have gone over some basics in "Scary Questions" it is time to "zoom out" to access a more psychological maneuver. What is it you offer your potential clientele that the business/person across the street can't? That isn't rhetorical. You're going to have to figure that out. I can guide you on specific models or options, but ultimately it's your personal skill set that is going to accentuate the avenue you choose to differentiate yourself. Earlier I touched on individual skill sets and how they tie into your fitness approach.

FIT Styles

For the sake of ease, our teaching style will fit into just two categories; Demonstrative and Direct-based.

Demonstrative: Focuses on mind/body connection, and fun before fitness/health. Most plans/regiments/workouts are based on the clients or classes immediate needs for that hour. Social aspect overrides physiological.

Direct: Emphasis on the goals, movements, processes, physiology/kinesiology, form, and typically a perfectionist. More likely to preplan and write out workout. Physiological aspect overrides social.

We are all hybrids of these categories, but finding out which style is more representative of you will give you a leg up on choosing your next steps. We are in the industry of helping people. There is a cathartic component to exercise and health that allows people to expel negativity through exercise or sport. Physiologically, our brains release endorphins, dopamine, and serotonin, but there is so much more which centers on clearing the mind from our "zoom out" psychological perspective. I have had hundreds of sessions in which the client preferred to vent to me about issues or concerns in their lives, personal or otherwise, rather than actually exercising for the 60 minutes of their paid time. I pride myself on making connections in order to be there for them in these situations, and never hesitate to do just that. Regardless of which teaching type you lean toward, you will have to deal with this and should do it happily. However, if this is somewhat concerning as you fall more into the "direct" FIT category, there are no shortages of options, so don't be concerned. For example, assessments or program developing allow you to focus on your craft and spend less time in personal discussion. There are also specific fitness routes where you can set your focus purely on body issues (e.g., NASM Corrective Exercise Specialist), thereby giving you the approach to be more physiology oriented, and not have the pressure of creating an experience or being the mental coach.

These two teaching styles always need to be fused together, but most of us are more one than the other. You have to know your skill set and play to it. People will seek out one of these two, expecting you to be stronger in one skill than the other. I already have a background in martial arts, and typically a tightly packaged daily schedule so when I take boxing lessons (as the trainee), I look for someone who is a highly-direct FIT to teach me. Those 60 minutes are at premium for me and are all about learning and improving my skill set through higher level techniques that I want to get from them. I do not chat and give off an obvious vibe of seriousness. Conversely, as a trainer I am more demonstrative, and attract that clientele. If an 83-year-old woman who has bilateral hip replacements, arthritis, and limited movement function of her upper body is coming to work with me, I'm positive it's because I am 60/40 demonstrative to direct. It could be, and likely is, the only 60 minutes she gets out of the house that day, and it's unlikely she is training to become a 100m sprinter, and more likely she needs the social component more than the technical. *Understanding your clientele and <u>balancing teaching and talking</u> is imperative.*

Niche/Specialties

Below are examples of niches in the fitness industry, and their sister sub-niches that are all too important to glance over.

Personal Trainer	Corrective Exercise Specialist
Yoga Instructor	Vinyasa outdoors
Group Fitness Instructor	Senior TRX Group Instructor
Life Coach	Women over 40
Health/Wellness Coach	Women pre/post pregnancy
Sport Specific Coach	Lacrosse speed/strength

You want to be a generalist who has a specialty. Okay STEVE, that is a contradiction! It sounds like it (and is), but let me explain further:

You can go to a Mixed Martial Arts (MMA) gym/school and learn all the different mediums of MMA. Wrestling, kickboxing, boxing, Jiu-Jitsu, etc. This appeals to the broader range of the public, as you can attract people of all backgrounds. If you're an MMA instructor, you have a background in all of these mediums. However, chances are you have an absolute expertise in one of them. For the sake of this conversation, let's say kickboxing. Your generalist approach will allow you to teach all of the martial arts mediums and gain a large following/clientele base. You can teach general MMA classes to all ages, hold self-defense courses for women, hold boxing classes for seniors with movement disorders, hold strength and endurance classes for upcoming martial artists, and the list goes on. Those are all moderately-priced and you'll use your generalist skills pitch to get people in front on you. With your expertise in kickboxing, you can charge far more because you've already demonstrated that you are proficient in all areas, and people will be even more intrigued to work with you in your individual specialty.

You're a Weight Loss Consultant owning your own business, and you also sell shakes/supplements which is your true field of expertise and passion, you will be well rounded enough to give general advice concerning workouts, sleeping, and eating regiments for your clients, but you'll only offer your supplementation guide at an additional rate for premium customers.

You're a personal trainer, and you specialized in kettle-bell functional exercises because nobody else in your city or gym has done so. On top of your general day-to-day personal training for clients of all ages and issues, you give two private evening advanced classes for men and women aged 18-35 who are looking to build functional strength in a High Intensity Interval Training (HIIT) format they pay a premium for. You've now secured a niche as "the kettle bell guy" while still maintaining a day-to-day generalist approach.

You're a yoga instructor for a new Bikram studio that opened up near your house. You do the smoothest headstand of all the instructors, and many of your students have complimented you on it. You start an outdoor private morning class in the park that focuses purely on movements that work toward achieving that headstand. You only take cash and private classes are 4-6 clients at a time. They have to pre-pay and book one week in advance as you politely tell them you have a waiting list.

Now that I gave a few scenarios on how using your niche can set you apart as a FIT, I want to explain how you fuse your teaching style (demonstrative or direct) with your niche. This step can only be taken once there is a greater understanding of clientele. This will all culminate in the next chapter when we discuss just that. Prior to that, let me give you another brief example using myself. I will elaborate on the WHY next.

Example of myself:

Teaching Style	Demonstrative
FIT Subject	Personal Trainer/Group Fitness
Niche	TRX Suspension
Clientele	Seniors
Sub-Niche	TRX Training for Seniors

How did I fuse them? I decided to teach TRX exclusively to retired seniors. Why? This is where we need to "zoom out" and look more at the social side. Seniors are generally more inclined to work with demonstrative trainers as they are typically looking for a social interaction coupled with overall health and wellness. They aren't as pressed for time as someone working 9 to 5, so taking breaks to tell stories and being a bit loquacious isn't an issue. Most TRX suspension training classes are all ages or catered to younger clientele so I separated myself into a sub-niche for seniors, which allows them to feel comfortable with easier movements. This scenario can be changed around infinite ways by switching the variables; teaching style (demonstrative), FIT subject (Group Instructor), Niche (TRX), clientele type (seniors), to fit your particular strengths.

What would be a comparable approach if the teaching style was Direct rather than Demonstrative?

Rather than a more friendly/casual class setting where you would be expected to always be "on" with humor or energy, you could prepare weekly individual assessments for a 6-month weight loss challenge for women only. You meet with people for 30 minutes, find out their particular goals concerning weight loss, and have specific tangible assessment numbers. Record their numbers (weight, body fat %, hip/leg/waist measurements, etc.), give tips and suggestions on how to improve and assist in the weight loss process. You meet with them at a designated date down the road to re-assess, and charge them a premium flat fee with a small grand prize (certificate) at the end if they meet their goals.

Teaching Style	Direct
FIT Subject	Personal Trainer
Niche	Assessment Based
Clientele	Women
Sub-Niche	Weight Loss Assessment

Which Style Makes More Money?

I once worked alongside a very talented personal trainer & yoga aficionado; for the sake of anonymity we will call her Ela. She had spent over 30 years in the fitness industry learning techniques and theories from physical therapists, yogis, and even orthopedic doctors. I never met anyone who had such a command when playing anatomical sleuth. With any issue that a client presented, she had the rare ability to work backward and find the origin of that ailment. Her clients appreciated her hard work. With that said, she was abrasive by nature, lacked emotional intelligence, and flat out didn't respond to teamwork so she was not the ideal colleague.

Alongside that colleague was her psychological profile antithesis; again for anonymity we will call him Wes. He had 15 years training, coaching, class instructing, and managing in different health and fitness facilities. Wes was the center of attention and lit up any room he entered. His humor and kindness were envious if not communicable. However, Wes lacked the skill set of truly understanding the body (or the urge to). His workouts, although creative, had little success in helping people achieve their long-term fitness goals if they fell outside of weight loss or enjoyment.

Both of these FIT were successful from a fiscal stand point, even given their lack of all-around skills. How? They chose paths that fit their abilities. Ela focused on corrective exercise assessments, individual 30-minute Pilates sessions, and yoga classes. The assessments allowed her to show her expertise of the body and injuries, and the 30-minute Pilates sessions ensured that the limited time would push the focus purely on the workout, and yoga attendees do not typically speak during class as all the focus is on the instructor's cueing of the movements. Wes took on Private Group Training (PGT) for young mothers and senior chair classes. Because the demographic of young mothers typically come with little to no physical issues, Wes could focus on making the class fun, playing great music, and building relationships, while not being burdened with requiring modifications for injuries. The seniors who were all sitting down in chairs, "Sit Fit", were frankly happy just to be moving and social with their friends. The amount of exercises one could do sitting was limited but extremely safe, and for that class, exercise was secondary to being in a positive environment that Wes created.

Having your niche and teaching style down is just the start. Now we have to be able to implement them into programs. I am going to give you examples of what other successful trainers have done to separate themselves from the pack, yet still doing exactly what they enjoy by using their skill sets and environment to their advantage.

Lenny started training at a fitness center on a beautiful southern coastal island with six golf courses nearby. He noticed the golfers didn't have their own class or personal trainer. The light bulb went on above his head as he imagined and mapped out how he could fill that role successfully. He did his research on golf fitness, started teaching a free class to get people interested, then passed a TPI (Titleist Professional Institute) golf certification. Now, he exclusively works with golfers, charges more per hour than an average personal training session (because he shows himself as the authority of golf fitness). He also will play 18 holes daily alongside of the golfers and take notes on their swings and body mechanics. Not a bad gig, huh?

Carrie noticed, after working long hours, it's better to work smarter not harder. Upon investigating, she came up with the notion that a lot of the older women preferred a private class done at their speed. So, she decided to create a Group Program class called Women On Weights (W.O.W.). She only allows 10 women per class and runs it four times per day. Each participant pays a third of the average cost of a training session, but having 40 women in there each day means she is making a killing for just three hours' worth of work. She then allowed other trainers to copy her model using the name and exercises she devises and takes a percentage of each class they run.

Marianne is a Pilates expert on the highest level. She noticed at her facility that couples tended to take part in leisure activities together (tennis, golf, bike riding, etc.). Marianne decided to be the authority in couples Pilates reformer training. This way she could make double by already having a clientele base; she now doubles it instantly by always having a spouse or a friend be brought in to join. She also learned to network with personal trainers. If their clients wanted to focus more on breathing, abdominal control, and body awareness they would send them to Marianne. She would in return send clients over who needed strength training. Marianne has a waiting list as long as the day.

Cara was simply a fitness enthusiast who loved attending HIIT and Circuit Training workouts. She noticed there were no outdoor classes in her area. She started working at a gym and spreading the word about her ideal class, and let it be known she was going to implement it soon. In addition, she attended various classes around the city and networked, also pulling "pick up/throw away" ideas though shadowing three hours a week. After a few months, she started an outdoor HIIT Bootcamp that was so well attended she had to move it after the second week in to get more space. She does two outdoor bootcamps per day with an average attendance of 35 persons, and each pays $15/per person in cash.

These are all real, true life sample models that different people have implemented to become successful as a FIT. Throughout the rest of the book, you will get a better sense of how you can form similar business models. You'll be given techniques and strategies to gain clientele and grow your business.

Continue to ponder and identify your teaching strengths, and if you and others close to you would consider your skill set to be more in-line with the direct or demonstrative approach. Again, most of us are a hybrid which is great for obvious reasons. Also, begin to think about areas of your current expertise that can be put into a sub-niche. If you don't have one, think about things missing (in your current/potential industry, city, gym, etc.) that you could gain a stronghold over. There are always hotbeds for certain industries that are ahead of most areas. For example, in the U.S., Los Angeles and New York City will have new group fitness classes before the South. International large cities will have nutrition and workout fads that work their way to the U.S. typically 6-12 months after they take hold. Do some research via Google in your particular fitness/health genre and find out what is trending. The key is to go where people are looking, not to insist they look at you. If you think it's of interest to you, and you don't currently have a specialty in mind, it may be for you. In our chapter on marketing, I will discuss how finding trends and using that initial fervor for your short- and long-term benefits is vital. Now that you have a baseline understanding of these concepts, it will guide you in choosing a more direct path to success.

After coming to grips with your teaching style and investigating your potential niche/sub-niche, whether you have the education or certifications, you need to hit the ground running. It's time to start learning and networking through the process of shadowing.

Shadowing

When I started at my first fitness studio, I had to shadow/assist over 500 hours of Pilates reformer work before I was able to teach on my own. It was miserable, mostly because I didn't like Pilates. Also, because spotting 73-year-old women with limited colon control in precarious positions doing abdominal exercises lends to some back-end exhales. During the process, however, I learned about the business, people, niches, and exercises I still today use across all mediums. I find myself using terminology I learned in Pilates when teaching everything from Muay Thai to golf fitness. All fitness/sports/health mediums have applications, theories, protocols, and constructs that expand generally over many fitness genres. Take the position of a squat; from yoga to football, you will be in this position over and over. The techniques and teachings to get into one will vary, but understanding the basics allows you to cross disciplines without actually knowing the specifics on how that discipline teaches it. Chances are you have had some experiences in sports or fitness that give you crossover knowledge, so remember to call on that.

Shadowing is done in every profession, but more often than not it is a forced educational requirement rather than for purposeful learning. As a FIT, you will most likely not have to shadow. Choosing to not do so on your own, however, is a mistake. It is a MUST. I will break down the process and its importance into three categories:

General Learning: Other FITs will almost always take you under their wing and be happy to teach you what they have learned. It is in our DNA to help and teach as a FIT, and asking to learn alongside a professional in your area or even getting tips from someone online you admire is a must. The more bodies and equipment you can be around, the faster your confidence and skill set will take ahold. You need to see different types of people and environments in order to hone your craft. I made it a point to work with a trainer who had a clientele of an older population (65+) when I first started. I began to understand their issues medically and the challenges they faced day-to-day. It widens the mind and scope of your exercise skill set when you are forced to be creative, and/or watch others do so when faced with challenging scenarios. Inevitably, you are going to have clients who come into sessions or classes injured. Maybe they pulled their back in golf earlier that morning or slipped down the steps and sprained an ankle the night before. How you decide to adjust and what you choose to work on to avoid those issues is partly based on your experiences in having watched others.

It's also important to force yourself to use equipment or styles you're unaccustomed to; but don't be afraid to say, "I am not well versed in that yet". Keep your eyes open, and head on a swivel to take in what other professionals are doing. I always stole from the best trainers I knew, and would tweak those techniques, exercises, plans, and protocols to my liking. You will be able to learn new exercises, techniques, verbal cuing, and more to develop into your best version of a FIT. It also gives you time to practice what you preach. You can go over these things time and time again in your head and imagine how you would train or set up things if you were in the shoes of the person you are shadowing. By routinely mentally completing something that you will eventually give to your clients (health plan, exercise routine, etc.), you will be able to demonstrate with authority as it becomes second nature.

Pick Up/Throw Out: Regardless if you work for a gym, studio, club, or on your own, you run a fitness and health business as if you own it all. You are not just learning tricks and techniques of your specialty, but you are learning how to run a business. Scheduling systems, marketing tactics, payments structures (e.g., per class, per week, avg price/hr, etc.), peak and low hours (volume of people/time), retaining clients, assessments, filling systems, small and large group dynamics. These are just a handful of the day to day issues a FIT has to deal with. It doesn't matter what the business model is (outdoor bootcamp, CrossFit gym, health coach), you can still learn things you want to steal and things you want to avoid by shadowing a similar business model. There is no better creative fuel than to watch a business similar to one you have in mind work (and not work). It will empower you to imagine exactly how you would handle all situations, from equipment purchase to scheduling. How do you truly know if a 45-minute class is better suited for your teaching style than a 60-minute class? Better yet, which one is more profitable? Finding out how much people are willing to pay in your area, and where the particular demographic is that best fits your business is imperative and will start at this step. Investing your time into a facility in order to ingest all of the information you need to create your perfect business is vital.

Job Security/Networking: At 22, I was hired to work in public relations at a business that I interned at the summer before. I was the only male in the office; I had a knack for computers, IT, and everything else electronic. Nobody else cared, or had that particular skill set. The copy machine would break on a regular basis, the server would fail, and I was the only person who learned how to burn b-roll onto a DVD. Between being male (outlier), having them already investing time in me (interning), and having a skill set nobody else had (electronics), I instantly gave myself job security. I use the same tools in the fitness industry to land top-level jobs. Shadowing allows you to gain the upper hand in all the aforementioned ways, but none more important than having a particular entity invest time in you which fiscally handcuffs them. It would be irresponsible to not hire you as training someone else would take time, and potentially money, and plus you've already learned their ways at no cost to them.

Employee retention is key, and even as someone not hired officially you will be looked at in a similar light while working alongside the team. Shadowing also has psychological components of cognitive dissonance coupled with what I call the strategy of attrition. Cognitive dissonance arises when a person holds two thoughts that could potentially be contradictory, so they in turn convince themselves that one is the proper thought to avoid the contradiction. This comes into play when you want to be hired at the place you're shadowing. They once saw you as green, but because they invested so much time in you while teaching you what they perceive are the ideal ways (their ways), they eventually believe you're indeed supposed to be there and are no longer a rookie. The psychology behind it will almost always prove true. By not hiring you, they would have an internal conflict of contradiction from their efforts by already investing time and energy into teaching you. The strategy of attrition comes into play from the perspective of the clients, members, and the others who regularly frequent the facility. You begin to build a rapport with people after so many hours of being around the facility that those people expect to see you and have now connected you with their routines. Humans are so routine-oriented (especially people who are regular exercisers) that you gain leverage purely through being around a facility long enough. You have worn them down so to speak and have now become ingrained into the day-to-day fabric of the business.

Through your shadowing hours you will also begin to see what particular skill set you have (or can obtain) that is missing in the industry, city, or at your specific work place. Maybe the facility doesn't have any female TRX Suspension Trainer Instructors, or male yoga instructors, or CrossFit-certified teachers. Find something during your shadowing that sets you apart. You may find yourself explaining nutrition or particular Olympic weight lifting techniques often and get pigeon holed as the expert in that area…that's what you want. This allows you to gain leverage, just as I did by being the only person who could fix the electronics in my PR office, or the only male Pilates reformer teacher in my first fitness gig.

Lastly, you will begin to meet other people who are of the same make-up and have the similar interests as you. You will have access to clients and others in your industry who you will gel with and can help you in near or distant future dealings as a FIT. I eventually landed my ideal job while shadowing. A trainer was out sick, and I had to fill in to teach a TRX Suspension Training class. I had experience using the TRX suspension trainer, but not in a class environment. However, I watched dozens of classes from other instructors, and took classes all over town. This helped me mentally map out how I would structure mine down the road, and when put on the spot, I delivered. One of the women enjoyed it so much she mentioned to me there were positions open at a facility she frequently attended, which is still one of my current places of employment.

Your best avenue to access and assess all the potential jobs in your area, and what your niche may be is to swim with the rest of the fish. However, obvious as some of this may sound, other people are not doing this. They are fearful or impatient. The advantage of getting your foot in the door even through a few hours of weekly unpaid shadowing, before or after you are certified, is priceless.

4 - FIT BUSINESS TOOLS & STRATEGIES

In order to get to where the aforementioned FIT success stories are, you are going to need some tools. Leverage is key, and you must provide yourself with it. All you have to sell is your time. When you understand this, when you truly take that in, you'll be much more likely to make every hour count for you fiscally. Understanding the principles in negotiating along with a handful of other business tactics can help you with gaining clientele, acing your interview, making your day-to-day work less demanding, and much more. Of course, your goal is to help people as a FIT, but you still can do this by working smarter, not harder. There are tools to use once you have implemented the marketing strategies. These tools help you keep the clients rolling in after the marketing strategies create interest.

Nail the Interview

All of the steps after this section can help you with your interview process as a FIT. However, I consider this an important enough standalone subject to elaborate on first, as most people are ill-prepared for their interviews as a FIT. I have interviewed dozens of FITs over the years and have put together the ultimate interview guidelines. There is nothing as potentially nerve-racking in any industry as presenting in front of people who you assume know more than you do on a particular subject. Most interviews in the fitness and health industry center on you doing a demonstration of sorts for people who are extremely knowledgeable in what is also supposed to be your realm of expertise. Your future job most likely hinges on this mock class, speech, training, or coaching sessions going off without a hitch. Let's go over the steps to ace this.

Research: I touched on this in "Scary Questions", and again as part of "The Art of Negotiating", but to reiterate, you have to do your due diligence in researching the company, facility, and/or people you are going to be potentially working with. Everyone has their own perspective and bias on what is best. You do not need to conform, but you at least should know what not to say going into an interview as a FIT. For example, if you are interviewing at a yoga studio, you may want to know that they specialize in Hot Yoga before you harp on your beliefs concerning only exercising while fully hydrated. You can dig up great content from social media and company-specific websites that allow you to be a step ahead in knowing what they are looking for. It is also a good strategy to have a few rehearsed phrases mentioning something the company, facility, or person has done or continues to do that you enjoy. For example, the CrossFit box you're applying to teach for may have a contest for most pull-ups in a minute every other Saturday. When the time presents itself in the interview, complimenting them and expressing your admiration for their creativeness in the pull-up competition will earn you brownie points and show you're a good fit as you appreciate their structure and methods. Lastly, there may be specific certifications or criteria that all their instructors have. You can use this to your advantage regardless if you share their same credentials if you have the same or similar training, understand what principles they are looking for and know how to present and use the parlance they are familiar with. If you don't, you can preemptively strike and let them know you are trained in a different skill set, and believe you bring value by having a different approach and viewpoint. Understanding what angle they are viewing things from allows you to structure your mock class/training in a fashion that is advantageous for you.

Practice: This next step is not only helpful in acing interviews, but in becoming the best FIT you can be. I have two strategies that will absolutely help make you more confident and competent as a FIT:

- Equipment Exhaustion Exercise (E3) – Every day for at least two weeks prior to an interview, grab a piece of equipment in your particular fitness/health medium and do everything possible with it. For example, if you're a personal trainer, you might grab a resistance band. Hook that band to a bar, put it under your feet, whatever comes to mind. Get creative, and feel free to tape yourself, or write out everything. Do every exercise you can possibly think of using that one piece of equipment. Make sure to hit the entire body. This forces you to think critically, anatomically, and creatively — all areas you will be challenged with in an interview.

- Site Specific Study (S3) – Pick out one area. A muscle, topic, movement, etc. Unload all of your information on that particular subject either out loud or, preferably, written out. For example, if you're a health and nutrition coach you may pick carbohydrates. List everything you know that relates to explaining carbs. This allows you to see areas you may need to brush up on. If you're a group fitness instructor you may pick out a muscle, chest (pectoralis major/minor). Write out every exercise you know that involves the chest muscles. These exercises give great insight into strengths and weaknesses in your current knowledge and allows you to have recent recall on particular subjects when asked during the interview process.

Confident, Honest, Teachable:

- Even though the interviewer is good and thorough, there is still a high likelihood you will falter at some point. Interviewers like to see how the interviewee reacts when given a situation or question that can either not be answered at all (trick), or is above their level of knowledge. If and when this situation arises, it is imperative that you don't freeze, lie, become embarrassed, or angered. Simply saying something to the extent of, "I'm actually not familiar with that, I apologize, but I'd love to learn that", will get you far more praise. Ultimately, people want to know you're easy to work with, and are teachable. These qualities as a FIT when trying to work for a company or facility are more sought after than absolute knowledge. Be yourself, be confident, be honest, and show you're <u>teachable</u>.

Art of Negotiation:

The following is simply a list of items you should have a solid grasp on before you interview or start building your independent career as a FIT.

Prepare – Research trends, research the organization, anticipate what could be said, assess strengths and weaknesses, your preferred outcome, alternative outcomes if you have to negotiate, concessions, prepare for emotional reactions.

Build Rapport – Show you're trustworthy, competent, likeable, and you have aligned interests.

Bargain – Give and take process, everyone should be equally satisfied or dissatisfied with the outcome.

Conclude –Reach agreement, lock in promises.

Execute – Follow through on agreement.

If you're interested in unpacking this esoteric topic, I suggest Roger Fisher and William Ury's, "Getting to Yes". In it, they urge you to keep the following four key principles in mind when negotiating;

People – Separate the people from the problem.

Interests – Focus on interests, not positions.

Options – Generate a variety of possibilities before finalizing.

Criteria – Insist that the result be based on some objective standard.

I understand these all seem like cliché business closer terminology better set for a real estate broker, but you should have a brief understanding if for no other reason than to feel confident when having to negotiate. Whether it be with your clientele or your boss, you will be faced with circumstances and situations that will be decided by your negotiation tactics for your entire career as a FIT.

Design Evergreen Content for Common Concerns: You will need content of some sort that you can use over and over (tweaking only when necessary) to help gain authority on your subject while simultaneously providing generalized value quickly. I developed stretching routines complete with pictures and step-by-step directions for five different, yet common, physiological issues (lower back tightness, poor upper body posture, etc.). When prospective or current clients came to me to discuss one of the five issues, I simply emailed them the pre-made file. It ups your credibility, portrays you are organized, and demonstrates you're a veteran in your field. If you plan on running an outdoor stroller class for Mom's, you will get the same questions asked over and over such as, "Are the exercises safe? I am only X weeks post-partum," and "What kind of cardio will we be doing and how fast can I lose my baby weight?" Having an email or flyer already on hand that answers those common questions will save you time and energy. Additionally, any time you can dispel potential worries, you increase the likelihood of getting them to participate or say yes.

Create Exclusivity Through Perceived Time/Schedule Constraints: For instance, if you are a group class instructor you can do this by capping the total number of attendees in each yoga class. This creates a sense of urgency and people will jump to sign up quickly. Even when you are fresh into the business, never tell your prospective client that your schedule is wide open. Always make them feel as if you're doing them a favor by fitting them in, and that you are busy. Your time and efforts are limited to the hours in the day, and you have to treat each hour as gold.

You can use quality or quantity to help build your fitness business. If you decide to work with smaller numbers of people, you have to use limited availability and specifically-catered programs to your advantage and upcharge for that. If you decide to work in quantity, you find ways to fit as many people into as few sessions as possible. This will allow you to charge them each a price well under the value and yet make it a steal for them financially. Understanding that collectively it makes you a lot more money not capping the total number of people when using that format is important. Here are examples of each method:

Holly is a golf instructor who instructs children and young adults from 5-18 years old in 1-on-1 private sessions. She works from 3 p.m. to 7 p.m. each evening after school and has now decided she needs to work smarter, not harder. Her new goal is to work one hour each evening for the same amount of money. She marketed herself through all the local schools and dropped her price point 50% lower than every other golf instructor in the area. However, Holly doesn't do 1-on-1 sessions anymore, but rather four or more at a time in group sessions only. Although the price per golfer is 50% less, simply by having at least four she is now making 2x or more of what she would have in an hour previously. She can now make what she used to make in an evening in one hour, at minimum, and most likely a lot more. She understood that it benefited the parents who would want to save money and that the children as a younger demographic aren't as particular about 1-on-1 time. The children and parents who still preferred the private session were faced with the dilemma of changing instructors or staying with Holly in the small group setting and saving money. They almost all chose the latter decision.

Jason is a Speed & Agility Training coach who works with high school and college athletes. He has a full-time business doing this and works with people both 1-on-1 and in groups throughout the year. Jason wanted to have a more relaxed summer, so he designed an "8 Week Summer Speed Course" to enhance their 40m and 100m speed. He let it be known he only has room for eight people. He charges $1,000 upfront per athlete and promises the following: daily workouts, free shirt with his Speed Camp logo design, 24/7 availability to questions/concerns, speed improvement after eight weeks, and his PDF course with full instructions. Jason only meets with the eight athletes, three times a week for one hour each meeting while they otherwise follow their own program. Collectively, over the course of the eight weeks, he works 24 hours (not including the initial course development time which is evergreen for new clients), which comes out to over $330/person. Jason understood creating a result-oriented product that had limited availability and little need for his physical presence was the ideal way to increase revenue.

Give Yourself Away: You need to get in front of people. You can use hours you otherwise would not be getting paid to give yourself exposure by giving your time up for free (or cheaply). Don't think of this as giving away your best asset, but rather investing it to save time (and earn more) in the future. This is no different than spending money to fix a water leak so that you can save money on your water bill down the road and ultimately come out on top. You can do this through social media, free local assessments, and many other creative ways.

When I was struggling to gain clientele in my second year working as a FIT, I decided to use the time I wasn't making any money and give it away for free. "Steve, I thought you said time is the only thing we have to sell as a

FIT, and now you're telling me to give it away? Get your sh*t together, Steve!" Remember, this technique appears contradictory, but in order to sell your time, you first need to acquire clientele. You won't have to do this down the road, but it's a great way to start gaining clientele quickly when you're green.

I needed something that was vague enough to draw in ample amounts of people but personalized enough where I was providing value. Choose a topic/subject, but don't narrow it down too much. I went with sports. Okay, now what? Well, design a sports-specific assessment! I designed an assessment that looks like a test, with 10 different exercises/stretches and their corresponding rankings (e.g., Plank Hold Test – over 2 minutes = 100). Some of the exercises/stretches were areas the prospective clientele were certainly going to struggle with, and that is purposeful. At the end of the assessment I want the subject to feel as if they could have, need to, or want(ed) to have done better. This is where we show our expertise and sell our value in helping them on whatever sections they struggle in. Maybe you had a golfer who came in and showed poor trunk flexibility in the rotational assessment and wants to now work with you on flexibility. Maybe you had a gymnast who came in and showed knee valgus in the single leg squat assessment and now wants to work with you to correct that. This can be done a million different ways for any FIT by simply changing the key variables:

1. Topic (e.g., sport)
2. Assessment/Test Type (e.g., exercises, stretches, combo of both, tests, etc.)

The key sell to them: It's FREE! It also provides value in giving the prospective client information about their physical skill set (or lack thereof) that they did not previously have from someone who is an authority (you!).

The key sell for you: Exposure. Access to prospective clients who are faced with their limitations. Ability to sell your expertise to fix those limitations. Who better to fix something than the person who first pointed it out? Show/tell them snippets of what you could do, but don't give it all away. Make them want to book you.

Adjust & Adapt: Ford Motor Company executives look over the Q3 (third quarter) earnings and purchases and see that they were selling Ford Focus's at a 3x higher rate than Ford F-150's. Assuming the margins on F-150's are significantly higher for each one sold, what do you think their focus for Q4 would be? Some may think putting more marketing into selling F-150's, however that would be a huge mistake. You do not create a market, you find out what the market dictates and you adjust accordingly. You would put all your marketing and sales teams on pushing those Ford Focus's out the door as quickly as you can, understanding the return on investment from a margins standpoint is less, but the quantity being sold given the market trends are large enough to make up the difference. That same strategy can be implemented as a FIT.

Ultimately, you will wear a lot of hats throughout your FIT career as you grow and learn new techniques, certifications, and fitness mediums. Understanding what is popular, and what will attract people toward you is vital. You'll have expertise in areas, and you'll love teaching specific fitness modalities more than others, but the end game to your success will be building your confidence in teaching anything and being ready and willing to switch strategies on a dime.

Let's say you have been selling a line of nutritional shakes that have various options of flavors, calories, macro-nutrient profiles, and vitamins. Suddenly, the Keto Diet has blanketed the entire food scene. Is your best bet to continue to push your best-selling shake that has strawberries and bananas (sugar is not keto) galore in it? Or to pull a quick marketing switcheroo to your coconut milk protein shake that is keto-friendly?

You have been running an outdoor circuit training class for a year centered on using kettle bells and heavy weights. Suddenly, a fitness challenge sweeps across Instagram; Body Weight Blitz. Everyone is trying to AMRAP (as many reps as possible) pushups and jump squats in 2-minute bursts each (4 min total) and posting their numbers. Should you continue course full steam ahead with your kettle bell and heavy weight movements? Or should you design and promote your class (or some of your classes at least) as the ultimate catalyst for maxing out the "Body Weight Blitz" by using exercises that specifically help your push-up and jump squat endurance?

I think you know the answers here, and there will be various scenarios daily, weekly, or yearly that will present themselves in a similar fashion and call on you to make these marketing maneuvers.

Complete FIT Business Prerequisites

There is no one correct way to attack your fitness business from a marketing perspective, but there certainly are wrong ways. Understanding a few key principles of marketing and finance are vital; demographics of purchasers, market expansion, and market exit. Attacking these elements preemptively will allow you to map out how exactly you see your business from the inception of recruiting clientele to a potential end game of selling it or having it run on its own.

Demographics of Purchasers: This is the most important, and the least sought-after information from young FITs. The people who are willing to pay for your services are the people who need to be targeted. If you have an Instagram page of 15k followers, majority of which can fit into these categories: international, under 34 years of age, zero personal interactions, then you essentially have no market. Unless you have established yourself as an absolute authority in your realm/niche, you will not persuade the three aforementioned groups to purchase anything. Proven purchasers in the health industry are the following: working professionals (34+), personal interactions, and retirees. In a study done by IHRSA, a whopping 61% of the recorded club/gym personal training fees were paid for by people over the age of 34. If your goal is to convince people in their 20's to pay for fitness and health private sessions, good luck.

As a FIT, your goal is to provide value for your clientele. Subsequently, the pay must be commiserated with the value you provide. If the going rate in your area for a personal training session is $60/hour and you believe you are providing $60/hour worth of value, who is now likely to be able to pay for that?

The people who have the funds to pay for your services and believe that your time is worth it are who you are trying to attract. This falls back on some principles I discussed earlier in "Adjust & Adapt". You do not create a market, you find out what the market dictates and you adjust accordingly. How many 22 year olds have 60/hour to pay a personal trainer? How many 24 year olds are likely to be nervous about transitioning from downward dog into warrior 1 pose? Juxtapose that with a 63-year-old now. These are the two factors that need to be understood:

Who has the funds to pay an expert?

Statistics take from a Deloitte Insights review reveal that nearly 20% of baby boomers have investable assets over half a million dollars, and over 35% have more than $50k in deposits.

Who is likely to seek out an expert?

The older you are, the more prone you are to injury/health related problems, and in turn the more you'll need a FIT to guide you. This is not just a pitch to your prospective clientele as a FIT, but truly a fact of life. It becomes increasingly difficult to lose weight, get stronger, and be creative in the exercise/health/fitness realm as you lose balance, motor coordination, strength, bone density, hormones, and stamina, all while increasing the fear of falling and obtaining life-altering health issues/illnesses.

Who needs your expertise more: A 67-year-old woman who was just diagnosed with osteopenia, or a 27-year-old female who wants to go from 123 lbs. to 115 lbs. for a wedding? You can certainly help both, but the 67-year-old will typically stick with you on a weekly basis, is financially more secure, and is less likely to take your tips and run.

Understand Scalability

If you are training deconditioned individuals on an hourly basis to work toward running a marathon, you will only have as many hours in the day as you can work to make money and help people. However, by creating a comprehensive training guide called "Couch to Marathon", you can sell the same information on a larger scale while not having to worry about being present. This is easier said than done as you will need authority in your subject in order to sell to buyers for whom you are not with face-to-face. Additionally, understanding the complexities of Google analytics, SEO, online marketing and sales is a job unto itself. Simply having this concept in mind for the purposes of a potential future business model shift is all that is necessary.

On a day-to-day basis, you may find that you have clients with similar goals and comparable fitness levels. When this happens, you should start to think about combining clients into groups. Coaxing them to work together in a duet session achieves the following: allows you to open up another free hour, reduces the cost for each individual client (duet sessions are typically split cost of 1.5x a normal session cost, giving them a 25% cost reduction), and gets you more money for that hour.

Market Expansion

Without pointing it out directly, I touched on a few of these strategies in the real-life examples I provided on other FITs successes earlier. There are a few questions to ask yourself when assessing if this stage is currently something you need to implement:

What markets am I currently reaching?

What other markets exist for my services?

What markets are easier to reach?

What markets offer greater growth?

What are the niches or fad markets?

You can interchange markets with people, areas, or demographics. Answering these questions not only before you start as a FIT but continuously throughout your career will allow you to form a centralized targeted attack on who potential clientele for you are.

Market Exit

This does not concern most people, but it is important to think about now, as the foundation of your business may be built differently if you decide your end goal is to sell your business or are renting a facility.

If you are building your fitness business with the intent to one day hire people underneath you and then sell it off, you will need to brand it in a generalized way. For example, if you're a busy mom who has developed a Beach Cardio Dance class with choreographed moves, you can teach other FITs how to take this on for you. However, if you call it "Danielle Johnson's Beach Cardio", it becomes increasingly difficult to transition the business over to having other FITs teach in your place or even buy the business outright from you down the road. You'll have a website with your name branded on it, and potentially other associations. Be general in your branding if what you're selling is a concept rather than yourself.

Additionally, capital equipment and redundancy costs such as contracts with vendors need to be addressed before exiting. A gym owner I knew went bankrupt almost overnight. Her lease was not resigned due to the owner selling the property to Walmart. Within 30 days she had to find a new location. To move that much equipment in a short amount of time and fork out a large down payment was too much of a financial burden. She was forced to close down and sell all the equipment for pennies on the dollar.

The initial excitement of starting a health/fitness business can blind you from the weekly, monthly, and yearly costs, not to mention the possible moving or exit costs. I implore you to physically write out all the potential options you have and estimated costs if things go south so that you're ready for a problem should it arise.

Networking – Inner Circle

I have mentioned networking in passing throughout the book on a few occasions. I gave examples of FIT networking with others in their industry and explained how shadowing can lead to connections. I want to elaborate on how important this is for our industry.

You are going to be faced routinely with questions surrounding all topics of health. Your clients value your opinion; this, however, can be a double-edged sword. There is no doubt you will feel the urge to make suggestions because you feel passionately about a particular medication or diet plan. Please remember, your opinions, when not directly associated with your credentials, should always be paired with the proverbial asterisk.

Sports Medicine Doctors, Orthopedics, Physical Therapists, Coaches, Nutritionists, Dieticians, and many other branches from the tree of health & fitness will most likely be working in some fashion of overlap with your clients. Your understanding of how these other pieces fit into that puzzle; that your client's health is vital for you getting them to their goals.

Additionally, creating relationships within the health community allows you to gain more clientele. By reaching out to these professions you can create a networking inner circle of referrals. These referrals are beneficial and necessary for four reasons:

1. The referral to a doctor or health expert in your community conveys to your client that you are connected, and thereby an authority in your realm of expertise.
2. Upon receiving the referral, the health professional will keep you in mind to send referrals to you at a later time.
3. Not stepping on toes is important. References show humility, and your client will appreciate you not working in areas that are not directly your expertise.
4. Your specific degree/certification will have limitations and expectations attached to them. You are liable if someone's health is affected from a direct result of you straying from those boundaries.

Over my years training I have learned more about the body working in a synchronized fashion with physical therapists, other trainers, and doctors than I ever could have imagined. Part of being a great FIT is your continued education, and networking will guarantee that. In most cities, there are networking groups you can join. They will typically only have one or two of each profession involved and you'll meet weekly to share referrals. A simple Google search will help you can find them in your area. You can also contact people via online social media who you may follow or respect in the health industry in hopes they can answer your clients' questions when the topic is fitting. I prefer the old fashion organic route of stopping by a few local offices with good reputations to introduce myself, and let it be known I want to refer clients to them when needed. If they are not easily reachable due to a busy schedule, I simply take a business card from that office and email them. There is no wrong way to network; as a FIT just make sure you do it!

5 - DAY TO DAY: WHAT TO EXPECT AND WHAT TO KNOW

Assuming you are officially sick from of all the "zoom in" marketing hoopla from last chapter, I am going heavier with "zoom out" talk concerning your expectations day-to-day on the job.

-Understand growth and learning is a part of the day-to-day process
-Personal Responsibility: feel as if you are being observed every day
-Have a long-term endgame in mind (i.e. only teach 20 hours a week of duet agility training)
-Remember the marbles: every insight and situation will help you become an expert

Build Your Reputation – Multiple Site Strategy

Ultimately, word of mouth is still the best marketing tool in our business. Even if you're growing your business with a social media focus, you're going to need reviews to get you noticed. Reviews are not fabricated, they are truthful, electronic versions of word of mouth marketing.

Before a parent chooses a pediatrician, before you select a dentist, or even before picking out a caterer for your New Year's Eve bash, what is it that we do? We find ourselves reaching out to friends and family for their advice or experience with the professionals in that industry or we jump on an online forum.

If you get a certification, and the next day you spread the word online, you're ready to do coaching calls with them, and they are taking a huge risk.

You are green to the market, and everyone knows that. You have to build your worth through learning locally and doing it at multiple sites. Why is the multiple strategy best?

1. Create leverage as a newbie: If you can start shadowing/working at multiple sites, you already have earned a sense of clout in the industry by people knowing more than one business was willing to take a risk on you. You will be able to bring tools to the table from each place and create leverage as eventually one of the places will most likely want to hire you full time, to take value away from the other competitor.

2. Different angles: You'll need to see things from different vantage points. Learning different teaching strategies from other FITs and business methodologies will help develop your sense of the perfect business style fit for you in the fastest manner. This also allows you to not only network with more people, but different types of people as every studio, facility, and gym will have a different demographic.

FAIR - Forms, Assessments, Insurance, Records

Always remember FAIR when starting with new clientele. When first meeting with a prospective client regardless of your health profession you will need some form of a PAR-Q (physical readiness questionnaire) and/or a health history form. You can find these online. Upon the client filling out the form, it is important you review it on your own first before meeting with them. There may be physical issues or medications you are unaware of and need to do your proper due diligence on prior to sitting down with the prospective client. If you feel uncomfortable working with someone who may have ailments above your current level of knowledge in order to make the proper exercise modifications, you should not work with that individual. This is where your networking comes into play as you should have knowledge of someone else who would be better suited to work with them.

When I meet with my clients in our first consultation after reviewing their health history form, I still allow them to talk as much as possible. Doctors sometimes call this the "what else?" session. If you continue to ask "what else" you'll be surprised to find the issues or ailments the client has or has had that they decided not to list on the sheet because they believed they were not relevant. For instance, if they broke an ankle 30 years ago, they are unlikely to write that down on a health history form. However, there could be compensations such as foot pronation, knee valgus, or pelvic twist accompanied by false leg length discrepancy, just from something as simple as a broken ankle at the age of 17.

Although I am a corrective exercise specialist, I do not always enjoy playing what I call "anatomical sleuth", so it is important to understand all of your clients' past injuries before doing your first assessment on them. It doesn't matter what your client's particular goals are because there are always ways in which you can do an initial assessment and track progress. This helps your client from a motivational standpoint, and it helps you understand what is actually working with your program. If weight loss is their goal, an obvious initial weight, measurements of specific body parts, and body fat measurement are in order (for body fat percentage I prefer bioelectrical impedance machine which you can get for $60). If you are unfamiliar with general assessments, I urge you to start reading up on all the various tests (Shark Skill, Rockport Walking, Step Test, etc.). You can also simply make your own up. I like to have my clients hold a plank until failure and find the weight they can get close to on 20 reps set for each of the following: low row, chest press, and leg press machines. This allows me to gauge their overall strength levels in core, pushing, pulling, and legs provided the clients goals and current health status align with that type of assessment.

Your company may provide you with insurance, but it is very cheap to double up and protect yourself. I do not recommend any particular company at this time, but the pricing should be between $8 and $15 per month. If you're training in home clients, or even at a park and an injury occurs you could be liable. In this age of overly litigious people it is best to always play it safe. You can do your own Googling to find out which company gives you the best rates.

Record keeping is important for both insurance reasons and your clients' overall goals. To cover the former, understand that if an injury happens and you are being litigated against from a safety issue, having records of what you did that day or week could save you. For the latter, you want to check progress from days, weeks, months, or years passed; having records allows you to do that. For a FIT who prewrites out the workout this is easy. I personally do not write out my workouts, so I have to make notes in my calendar (Google calendar is where I keep all my sessions) if there were any issues that day as far as slips, slight injuries or tweaks, etc. Cover yourself. Keep records.

Intellectual Curiosity

<u>Don't be afraid to both learn and bounce your ideas off others in and around your industry.</u>

As a personal trainer we do not diagnose injuries, but it's important to know that there are tell-tale signs and tests. Imaging is typically needed to truly be accurate, but the tests and signs give high probability indications of the issue existing. What is not as clear however are the treatment protocols for the issue. Even as a corrective exercise specialist, I sometimes find it difficult to play anatomical sleuth and decipher what issue to treat first and how. For instance, if you're a FIT you've likely heard the term IT band. The iliotibial band extends from the iliac crest (hip) down the lateral part of the thigh a few inches above your knee to the distal lateral femur, and then part of it connects lower past your knee cap to your proximal lateral tibia and provides stability to the knee and assists with flexion and extension of the knee. When clients have knee, hip, or low back pain, the IT band is a check point of sorts to determine whether that is the culprit. Is it the IT band causing knee issues or the knee issue causing a hip issue, which is in turn causing IT band issues? You can have IT band syndrome, or Greater Trochanter Syndome and a host of other issues due to issues with the IT band. It is a very esoteric subject and I have barely scratched the surface, so for the sake of this topic we won't unpack the anatomical specifics anymore.

However, when dealing with potential IT band issues, I've had physical therapists tell me you cannot stretch the IT band because it's a tendon and it doesn't get tight, and that it's hip weakness and glute strengthening that you should be treating more often than not. I have had sports medicine doctors disagree with that assessment and prescribe specific stretching routines and rest for those areas. I have had personal trainers I respect confidently relay that it's typically overworked rather than tight, and myofascial release is the fix. None of these statements are outright false.

There are different means of treating the same ailment and complexities specific to each case.

Learning different methodologies and being intellectually curious in your field of work is important. You will have clientele who come to you and may have worked with other FITs in the past. Those professionals may have instructed movements different than you. Their educational background can affect the way they cue and explain movements. There is a gray area in the fitness world, so don't assume without doing your due diligence that the one way you've been taught is the only way.

Working with challenging populations can further instill the urge to attain more information from other professionals. Even if the niche you work in is with a younger population who typically have no serious medical issues or limitations it is still best to have some experience with a more challenging population. It will take away standard exercises and make you think outside the box for modifications and force you to get better at simplifying and being creative.

Protocols and routines will always change, depending upon the individual FIT and their educational or historical background. It is important to continue to learn in order to stay ahead and in line with the thoughts of current medicine and health perspectives. In the past, personal trainers recommended static stretch before exercising, and now the science tells us dynamic stretching prior to exercise is preferred and static stretching is more advantageous post exercise. Some science even tells us people who are already hyper flexible don't need to continue to stretch on a regular basis. The point is, you can find differences of opinions, but the important concept is the approach to the patient should always be the same; keeping their best interest in mind using the knowledge and skill set you've acquired. Learning from others who are in the same field, but have different approaches is important to challenge the way you interpret issues and help you grow. You will more than likely start off conservative in your approach to any fitness medium. As you continue to learn, you will find yourself gravitating toward specific teaching styles or modalities, and some may even be radical. Eventually most of us come back to the center as we gain more knowledge from all the industries that touch ours. Wherever your road toward greatness takes you, learning, researching, going to conferences, getting new certifications, and growing by conferring with other FIT and similar industry experts is a must.

Managing Schedules and Situations

You are going to have to learn to be a good secretary. One of the most potentially frustrating parts of your week can be scheduling. As a FIT, it is a great problem to have, being that it means business is good. However, this does become increasingly agitating due to potential over interest in booking during the "high times" and lack of interest in the "low times". Just like restaurants, clothing stores, and super markets, there are times of day when people are more likely the flood a particular business. For example, you don't go to the bank at 12 noon as you'll be in line for an eternity with everyone else in the area on lunch break. I never understood why aren't banks open from 6 a.m. to 9 a.m., and then again from 4 p.m. -10 p.m., when people are out of work to be more accessible? I digress. Filling midday spots is typically more difficult for personal trainers. People who work 9 to 5 are likely to come before and after work, yet even business owners and retirees are less likely to come midday. Would you want to wake up, shower, get dressed, run errands, change into gym clothes midday, exercise, shower again, get re-dressed and go on with your day? Finding clientele who are willing to fill the times less sought after is key. Some of this is purely luck based on people's schedules; however, you can use some scheduling techniques to aid in this:

Price adjust: If you control the pricing of your business, you can drop the price for what you deem "low interest" times. This will certainly help fill those slots.

Exclusivity: We talked about this previously. People can, and will, adjust their schedules for what they deem important or worthwhile. It's not just about the value, it's also about the story. People are willing to pay more for Nike shorts even if they aren't made of anything different material wise that would suggest they should be more valuable than Russell Athletic. If you built your brand and established yourself as a professional for whom people admire and respect, they will pay more for your services or be willing to accommodate your schedule. When you're trying to fill slots and talking schedules with new and prospective clients, learn to lead with suggestions: "How about 11 a.m. on Monday and Wednesday?" rather than say,

"Whatever works best for you!!". Emphasize that you have limited availability, and they will try to fit into your schedule.

Scheduling Programs

There are a host of scheduling programs one can use for any appointment-based fitness business, big or small. Schedulicity, Motionsoft, Glofox, Vagaro, and MindBody are the ones that come to mind. If your business simply consists of you, booking sessions for yourself, I would stick with Google Calendar or your choice of something similar. There is no reason to add bells and whistles and pay for scheduling programs. If you decide to let clients (or classes) book on their own, then I would recommend all the previously-mentioned programs as your best options. You can limit class sizes, block off specific times/hours, have multiple employees' schedules listed, and even charge your clients through these applications. I don't have any affiliation with these programs, but from my personal experience I would recommend Vagaro for people working 1-on-1 sessions, and MindBody or Schedulicity if you're more class oriented or plan to have multiple people working alongside/under you. You can use free trial versions for most of these, so I would do your due diligence before purchasing.

Simple Do's and Don'ts When Working With Clients

While on vacation in Miami, I was getting a personal morning lift in at a local gym. I couldn't help but to glance over at other trainers to see what sort of experience they were providing. There were only two trainers working at the time in a relatively small gym consisting of five treadmills, a handful of machines, kettle bells, and free weights. Both trainers were in great shape, in their mid-30's, one with blonde hair the other with brown, and seemed to be working for the same independent company as they were wearing t-shirts that said something to the extent of "NAME'S Fitness". For the sake of this story I will call them Trainer Blonde and Trainer Brown. Trainer Brown's client was on the treadmill as he strolled in at 8:21 a.m. Her eyes rolled and a half smirk arose over her face as he slowly walked toward her apologizing, "The line was super long at Starbucks, my bad", sipping his coffee. After already arriving late with a coffee in his hand, he then proceeded to ask his client, "What do you want to do today?". Trainer Blonde was across the room working with his client, a women in fabulous shape somewhere in her early 40's, 5'5" 125 lbs. Trainer Blonde was having her do dumbbell deadlifts. He didn't instruct form, tell her how many repetitions to do, or ask her anything outside of, "Can I film you when you do these? It will be great for my website?"

I couldn't help but be angered by this. How do these guys have the same job title as me? Why would anyone ever work with them and pay good money to do so? My guess is that they both had a very small overall clientele base, and may have been out of work by the following week. Regardless, it's a shame.

Over the years I have become both sickened and occasionally laughably in hysterics when watching mistakes FIT make while working with clients. Most of these do's and don'ts boil down to one thing: The Golden Rule. People are paying money for your time and expertise, and you have to treat them as you would expect to be treated. I will go over a simple list of things to keep in mind so that you always appear to be engulfed and focused on creating a positive experience for each client.

1. *Be early, not on time* – other potential clientele are always watching, always. At least half of my clientele had watched me work in some capacity from afar or were told via word of mouth about my professionalism prior to working with me. You are a professional. Don't ever be late. Additionally, you need to assess the layout. Whether you're teaching a class or working one-on-one with someone, showing up early allows you to see what equipment is available (or not), any issues there may be with the facility (air conditioner out, treadmills broken, etc.), and allows you to make any last second adjustments in your plans so that any curveballs that may be thrown your way do not cripple your ability to put together a good experience. Imagine if I asked you to put together a routine for me (any fitness medium) using three different items in a place you are familiar with. Now, imagine I dragged you into my facility and asked you to do the same thing. You will spend half of your time looking around the space to find items you thought of in your head that you had exercises for. It makes you look unprofessional and shakes your confidence. Understanding the space around you is a must, and being early allows that. Thinking

on the fly and being creative is important and inevitable, but having one leg up will make that easier.

2. *Ask your client how they feel – I call this the "Update".* This should always be the first question you ask. You need to check in with them physically and emotionally. Letting them vent for the first few minutes of every session gives you solid direction as to what type of experience you may need to provide, or what exercises you should avoid. For example, if your client tells you they worked out on their own and ran 12 miles the day before as they are training for a marathon, it may not be best to structure your workout around leg exercises that day. You may need to reassess your game plan and put together a lighter workout focusing on upper body, core, coupled with dynamic and static stretching. Be prepared to receive a host of different responses such as, "I didn't sleep well last night", "I have had some stomach issues", "My gout is flaring up", "I'm just upset about some things going on with my partner", "I feel really fat today", and everything else under the sun. You have to be ready to pivot and adjust to their needs. It also allows you to go over their goals and reiterate that you know where they want to be and that you're helping them stay on track.

3. *Come prepared –* when I previously wrote about Trainer Brown asking his client, "What would you like to do today?" you may have thought, "What's wrong with that, Steve?" It's only wrong if it's the first question you ask. You want to show your client or class you already have a plan in mind, and that you've come to work prepared. After asking them how they feel, and getting their response, only then should you give them an option of choosing what to do. Yes, they are paying for the session and you should provide them with whatever services they specifically ask for. But that doesn't let you off the hook from coming prepared and emphasizing that you are the FIT with the tools that are helping them toward their goals. Using online forums is something I highly suggest as a resource to pull great exercises from. Of course, you should always take anonymous online posts with a grain of salt, but there is a lot of great information and routines you can pull from to help guide you when writing out a plan.

4. *Demonstrate & Elucidate –* your ability to demonstrate and elucidate needs to be on display continually. For a few of the same reasons I have previously mentioned, prospective clients are always watching, and you need to illustrate that you are an authority and expert in

your realm. It is also the safest and easiest way for your client to learn properly. Whether they are visual or auditory, you are covering both bases as far as proper form is concerned. People also like to see things done with ease, in an impressive manner. They should be enamored by your skill set in showing the movements, which reemphasizes why they are paying you. You should also be elucidating the "why" for movements so that you again show there is a purpose and a plan, additionally illustrating your ultimate understanding of the fitness subject. People learn in a variety of ways. You have to learn to be adept in explaining the same thing in various ways. For example, when putting my client into position for a rotational exercise I have different terminology I will use until something clicks. I may say, "Get into an athletic stance." If that isn't enough, I can get more specific and say, "Pretend you are playing second base and anticipating a ground ball." Understand that what is easy and normal terminology for you will not be for your clients. Be ready to try different phrases, analogies, and visual stimuli.

5. *People Learn Differently* – it is your job to be good at presenting things in different ways until the client understands. You must use different visual cues outside of anatomical parlance in order to get people to understand the movements and connect the dots. For example, when describing the kinetic chain progression of a squat, it is typically much easier to say, "There is a door open behind you I want you to pretend you are going to push the door closed with your butt before you start your squat," rather than, "Hip hinge backwards into an anterior pelvic tilt position." Remember that your clients do not understand (nor care) about all the specifics, and they rely on you to put them into the proper positions by relaying that information to them in whatever way is easiest for them to process. Many times, you will have demonstrated each movement as some people learn from the visual stimuli. Have at least three ways of demonstrating or describing each of the Central 7 Movements (which you will learn shortly).

6. *Quick & Confident* – you know that feeling when you're about to watch someone in a horror film walk into the room where the killer is? I get that same wide-eyed discomfort when I watch trainers drag their clients around a fitness facility, aimlessly looking for an idea or an exercise to pop into their heads. The equipment isn't instructing you what to do, you're using the equipment to help instruct your client. If your internal monologue is always churning

from an anatomical perspective, "We've worked legs, core, and pulling…okay let's do pushing next," then you can be proactive in getting to the next exercise swiftly and confidently to show your client you have a plan. Once you understand the "Central 7", which we will go over next, you should never have an issue with this.

Understand the Central 7 Movements

This section is a "zoom in" directed at personal trainers and group fitness instructors, but can truly help anyone in the health & fitness industry if you take a step back and "zoom out" to adjust it to your fitness/health medium. Every sport, exercise modality, and general subject has a foundation. Understanding and branding these movements deep into your brain so that you never forget them will ensure that you never run out of creative exercises to offer your clients. The following are the Central 7:

(If you are new to personal training, do not be overwhelmed by some of the more kinesiology-based terms. Simply understanding the pictured movements allows you to be creative, and learning the physiology can come at a later time.)

Plank: Neutral spine, level pelvis, alignment of ears, shoulders, hips, knees, and ankles. Everything is stable, and nothing is mobile in a standard plank.

The focus is on maintaining tension while keeping stable.

Core strength is the focus here, and it translates to almost any exercise or activity. It is the basis and bedrock strength for all other exercises to be done correctly without compensation or synergistic dominance.

Push: Proper alignment of scapulohumeral (shoulder blade & arm) ensuring optimal positioning for pushing force. Core activation and proper alignment of the spine are vital here. Keep the lower body stable as you move the object(s) away from center mass.

Also known as pressing, the shoulders, chest, and triceps are the main muscles activated here while your core is braced, and the movement occurs.

Pull: Holding a neutral spine while bracing your core is what is called an "active plank". Maintain that position while moving the object(s) toward your center mass. Keeping a consistent speed, focusing typically in scapular retraction and depression (shoulder blade squeezed, lowered).

Pulling emphasizes larger back muscles as the prime movers and uses the arms (such as the biceps) and the smaller muscles in the back (such as the rhomboids) as synergists.

Lunge: Front foot flat, rear foot using the ball of foot to stabilize while maintaining a tall spine. 90-degree angles for both legs. Rear leg shin parallel to ground. Front knee directly over ankle, and back knee directly under hip.

Emphasis on equal weight distribution, and tall stable spine and mobile knees, ankles, and hips.

Glute, quad, and hamstring activation. Bipedal motion mimics walking and running.

Squat: Straight spine, begin from hip and knee extension and descend to hip and knee flexion until your hips are right above your knees. The angle of your belly button to neck should be the same as the angle from your ankle to your knee.

Focus on slight outward pressure on the feet to ensure zero knee valgus (inward dip) and recruit maximum amount of leg muscles.

Local core stabilizers, quads, glutes, hamstrings. Squat is one of the best exercises to evaluate a client's compensations and limitations.

Rotate: Moving through what is called the transverse plane, anything from the toes to the head can be shifting in a cylindrical fashion. Anything from a golf swing to a Russian twist fits under rotation.

Emphasis is typically on thoracic spine movement, with minimal to zero (unless highly controlled) movement below the waist. Often the goal is lower and upper body disassociation, meaning we move them separately.

Core strength is a key as the ability to use or let go of the brace technique is vital, but proprioception and speed are also valued in this range of motion.

Hinge: Holding a neutral spine, while moving from hip flexion to extension while simultaneously moving from a slight knee flexion to extension.

Hip drive is the emphasis here, while maintaining neutral spine and relaxing upper body appendages.

Lower body and torso muscle groups engaged, particularly posterior chain.

Now that you have an idea of the Central 7 movements, it is time to unpack how you can use a handful of variables to give you endless creativity in movements for your clients.

D.O.T.S

D.O.T.S is an acronym I created to help you quickly recall four important fitness factors to stay creative when working with clients or classes; **D**uration, **O**bjects, **T**empo, **S**tability.

Using D.O.T.S and fusing together Central 7 movements will give us endless exercise options, and the ability to think quickly. First, decide which one of the Central 7 movement types, or combinations, you are going to focus on. Then pick out any exercise that comes to mind and put it into the D.O.T.S formula. For example, let's choose "Squat" from the Central 7, and *Front Squat* as our exercise;

Duration – 90 seconds

Object – 20 lb barbell

Tempo – 2 seconds up (concentric/positive motion), 2 seconds down (eccentric/negative motion)

Stability – Normal width-base, feet on ground

Through repetition, you can get your mind to always wander to D.O.T.S right after you decide your Central 7 movement, and particular exercise. Continue to change any of these variables to fit your clients' needs provided it's in a safe manner in order to keep your routines creative. Let's use the same exercise for a client who may be more seasoned in weight training:

Duration: 20 repetitions

Object: 70 lb barbell

Tempo – 1 second up (concentric/positive motion), 3 seconds down (eccentric/negative motion)

Stability: Standing on a Bosu Ball

Just to reiterate:

1. Choose one movement from the Central 7 movements (e.g., Push)
2. Pick an exercise that fits into that category (e.g., Bench Press)
3. Use D.O.T.S to decide how the exercise will be completed (e.g., D: 10 repetitions, O: 45 lb Olympic Bar, T: Explosive Concentric, 2 second eccentric, S: Standard bench position.

Booking 9-5 Evening Clients

When you're working with people who have busy schedules, you have to ensure that both old bad habits are squashed, and newer better ones are developed. Habits are automatic responses to triggers. If you come home and go straight to the couch and put the TV on, you will continue to do so until you change the habit/trigger. Given their lack of free time, they are going to pick one of three time periods: Before work, lunch, after work. I think the first two are always the better options for the above-mentioned reasons.

Choosing what time of day is best to exercise is important. There are both physiological and psychological components that need to be addressed. If after work, exercise is ultimately the chosen option, you'll have to stay conscious of the following three factors: energy, exercise intensity, gym proximity.

Energy: In the nutrition world, calories and energy are synonymous. However, we know sleep, mental exhaustion, insulin spikes, nutritional habits, vitamins, and other variables play a role. You will have to make sure your clients are close to optimal energy by the end of the day. Many take supplements such as "pre-workouts" to negate the fatigue from a full day of work. However, if you're a personal trainer, you are not in the business of recommending supplements. You can recommend when they eat (without what). Everyone's body is different, but through trial and error you'll have to guide them to find the right foods, and teach them the right times to eat so that you're not going to get a client who is exhausted, full, or both!

Exercise Intensity: With all that said on energy, sometimes the gas tank is simply empty. Maybe they've had a tough day at work trying to cram and meet deadlines that were pushed up. They have a mind and body now both completely exhausted. This is where they actually need the exercise to decompress, and get some endorphins flowing, but most people will find excuses to get on the couch and Netflix binge. You need to pre-plan by having "light", "moderate", and "intense" days, and choose the type of workout to use according to their energy level. Again, everyone's body is different, and your goals will lend toward specific workouts (e.g., weight loss, marathon training, muscle building, etc.). Regardless, understand what exercise mediums your clients enjoy the most, and what may be more difficult so that you can revert to the type that corresponds to their energy level on that given day. For example, 45 minutes on the elliptical "climb" program may be light for your client. Conversely, 30 minutes of a Kettle Bell training may be very difficult.

Gym Proximity: When working with clients who meet me after work, I find out where they work, and what time they get off, and set the appointment for the exact time it takes to get to the fitness center from their office. Why? In my 10+ years personal training, I've noticed a reoccurring theme; stopping home increases your likelihood of not working out 2x fold due to the bad habits I touched on earlier. They will always find something at the house that needs to be done. You'll open the fridge and notice you're out of milk, you'll have messages on your phone you need to return, you'll remember you're hosting a dinner Friday and haven't washed the tablecloth. Instill in them that they must make exercise their priority and get them to always be prepared to go straight to the fitness facility, track, boxing gym, etc., right after work.

Long-Term Motivation

Understanding motivation is an important factor when first working with clients. Motivation comes in all different forms. For the ease of this particular conversation, let's break them down into three major groups:

Vanity: many people tackle fitness/nutrition through vanity and have a particular goal of looking a certain way; this may be self-esteem based, or simply trying to get back to size, strength, or shape they once had. Vanity is a great motivator. Do not discourage people from using this as their motivator unless you deem it unhealthy. Even in those cases, be cautious to avoid judgment and direct them to speak with someone who is suited to handle a potential eating disorder or something of that ilk. A good way to keep this as the motivator but to combine it with a healthier component is to do measurements. Clients will get fixed on the scale solely. Having more initial baseline reference points will give you a better opportunity to point out the positives. For example, if you do initial body fat % measurements, hip, waist, mid leg, lower leg, arm, chest/back, and weight, you can point out which points are going in the right direction when you re-measure to check progress. If you only record their weight, you have a 50% chance they are going to be upset.

Competition: Many former athletes, or naturally competitive people find races (e.g., 10k, marathon, etc.) 90-day programs, or friendly bets with family to be the motivational driver behind taking the first step back to a healthier lifestyle. This allows people to visualize their goal and keep constantly aware of the ramifications of deviating from the healthy patterns. The competitive drive pushes them toward healthier choices, including hiring a FIT. If you have clients who use competition as their motivator, be prepared to design workouts that are goal oriented, as well as monthly or annual markers to reach.

Health: Others take a more total body health-based approach and focus on things such as lowering cholesterol, dropping total body fat percentage, and increasing energy/mood. Anyone who has gone to the doctor after their yearly labs only to be scolded for their numbers, understand this scary rude awakening. Realizing that your overall health is on par with someone of the same age, and that your future quality of life will be affected can be plenty of motivation to kick start a proper diet and exercise routine. If this is your client's motivational driver, you may ask their permission to see their labs or simply be passed along the information (from them) that their doctor has given them. Learning how to read a basic lab panel reports is easy, and necessary in my opinion to set yourself apart from the average FIT. Your client will be impressed with your ability to understand their health on all levels.

Understanding which of these (or combinations) are your clients' motivational drivers is essential for not just creating a plan but for developing a bond and keeping them on track.

Short Term Motivation

People are going to have bad days and weeks, and part of your job is to keep them on track with their goals and get their mind in a better place. Mixing up workouts is a great way to do this and a must for your tactical arsenal. Let's say for instance you are training someone who wants to run a 10k. You've been working together for three weeks, and the race is six weeks away. They are starting to think they won't be able to do it. Having planned six different workouts already, you assessed which workouts your client enjoys the most/least, and which ones are needed the most/least is part of your job. Below are the different training days for your client:

-Long Distance Indoor Running

 Long Distance Outdoor Running

-Ab/Strength Work,

-Slow Pace Run

-Stretch/Recovery

-Sprints/Speed Work

1. You can set the schedule weeks in advance which some clients if they prefer that structured style, or keep them guessing if you feel that is better for their personality. Keeping them on their toes and manipulating the schedule from week to week allows the over thinkers

to stay focused on day-to-day regiments.

2. It also allows you to psycho-analyze their needs and puts the appropriate workout at just the right time. If they are bored or frustrated with training, make sure you give them the day they enjoy and/or are best at. If they just need to talk something out due to external issues going on outside of training, it's a great day for a slow run and emphasis or put emphasis on stretching/recovery.

3. Lastly, it allows you to challenge them. They are going to be great at some of these (e.g., Indoor Running) and may struggle with others (Ab/Strength). Keeping them honest and understanding there is always more work to be done is a great way to stay on task.

When to End It

Although you can't be picky right away, down the road you are going to want to make your life easier by working with clients who you enjoy and appreciate you. You are essentially in a relationship and although behind every good relationship is hard work, some are doomed from the outset regardless of the efforts. So, you need to make sure that you fire clients for whom you do not care to work with. If those clients put you in a bad mood, it's going to affect the rest of your day and subsequently your relationship with the rest of your clients which will hinder your business collectively. You can try and be honest with them and have a conversation about issues you are having; however, this typically goes one of two ways: everything gets resolved and you become much closer with your client, or s*** hits the fan and you're dealing with someone who is ego driven and feels offended. If you decide to go the route of cutting ties, one way to do this is to simply only offer hours that you know are not doable for that particular client. For instance, you let them know that the only time you have available is 5:30 a.m. all the while knowing they are not morning people. You can also pump up one of your colleagues or fellow networked connections and tell your client how you feel that professional is better suited for their particular needs and pass them along. I typically choose this method, and it has never been a problem. A change is good, and I have given away clients in the past when I believe the situation has grown stale; and both parties were happy at the end.

Private Group Training (PGT)

PGT, also called Small Group Training, is a recent trend that has exploded in the industry. This is not specific to personal training as the format of having 4-12 people in a pre-scheduled format is a method used by all genres of FIT. *IHRSA's Profiles of Success* reports that 18 million health club consumers signed up for PGT in 2016, accounting for 26.6% of the total consumer base. **PGT participants are more likely to be female, but that's not surprising as almost all fitness-related attendance is.** Generation Z had the highest participation rate for PGT, which was thought to be over a quarter of their population (4.8 million).

In my experience, older populations are attracted to PGT. It allows them to have comradely, privacy, and trust that a good FIT will focus on low to no impact routines. Statistics from IHRSA claim that the 65+ senior group had the second highest rate for PGT market at 25%.

The advantages to this should be fairly obvious, but I will go over them in depth in order to not only provide you "zoom out" reasoning, but "zoom in" techniques to keep in mind, if and when you decide to jump into this format for yourself.

Pricing is the ultimate selling component here due to it being significantly cheaper in this format for your clientele, and conversely higher per hour for the FIT. The price point is lower than a personal training session which drives people toward it. In 2016, $34 was the average cost to participate in a PGT session, but multiply that by 4 to 12 and you'd be raking in the money. This is not a group class setting where people can show up and pay as they come. This is simply training or teaching of a particular type (yoga, personal training, Pilates reformer, Olympic weight lifting, nutrition tips) with a limited amount of spots, and premium charges paid up front. Your goal should be to provide as much, if not more, value than you do for a 1-on-1 session. Why else would someone pay double a class price for what is essentially a small class? You have to make the environment personal, fun, unique, and over the top. In the long run, even spending your own money out of pocket for the clients in these particular classes is a wise investment. I am going to elaborate on a particular trainer and the PGT I touched on before. This example will unpack the entirety of advantages and give you more of a tangible idea as to how you can structure something similar in your niche.

Carrie's W.O.W. was structured around helping women over the age of 60 feel comfortable and confident getting stronger using weights and other tools with the primary focus of strength training. She noticed during her day-to-day personal training sessions that a host of women entering senior ages were hesitant to join in standard strength classes. Upon investigating further, she found that: 1) Group class instructors did not always have adequate modifications to make them feel as if they were getting a great workout, 2) They were simply embarrassed having to essentially take a different class then the rest of the younger population due to all of the modified movements, and 3) They were fearful of falling and wanted to increase bone density while improving balance.

Realizing there was a need with senior women looking for strength training fitted to their level, Carrie began to develop a program specifically for them. She understood that this is typically a population who has money, and that they are willing to pay for a premium product. She charged double the price of what a standard group fitness drop in class would be, but that was still 60% cheaper than a personal training session. She advertised the class first through word of mouth telling a few women she already worked with that there were only a handful of spots open in the first few weeks creating exclusivity. She then created a flyer that emphasized 60+ aged women only, the small group exclusivity, the financial incentive compared to a 1-on-1 session, the focus of strength and balance training, and the environment of safely-chosen movements specific to fit the small group attendees.

After getting over 20 people interested, she sat down with each potential client for a 30-minute paid consultation on their health history as well as hopes or suggestions for what they'd like in the PGT. This gave Carrie a plethora of data and detailed information on how to structure the PGT, along with 20 paid consultations that made the potential clientele feel invested as partially their own. After assessing the information gained from the consultations, Carrie established the following preferences: Training times, exercise types, personalities, injuries, music, positive feedback, among many others. She did not however, discuss pricing as an option. Given that she could provide all of the requests and desires that she accumulated from the consultations, she felt as if a premium charge should and would be paid without any arguments or need to haggle. She had the attendees who were "approved" to take the PGT sign up for all the classes they planned to attend in the given month. They needed to cancel 48 hours in advance, or they would be charged. Establishing the pricing precedent upfront is key.

Before the first PGT, the room was pre-set up with names for each location and all the appropriate weights and fitness toys that corresponded to what she acquired from their individual goals and health history forms. There were women with movement disorders, knee replacements, shoulder injuries, etc. She was ready in advance with modifications or equipment specific to their needs. There were towels set up for each attendee along with water, and an energy snack called a W.O.W. ball (almond butter-based food she created for the class). She had a sheet with everyone's name, husband's name, pet's name, previous surgeries, health complications, occupations, college attended, and more. This allowed her to personally connect with everyone during the class, bringing up topics and questions centered on the information to make it a positive and fun environment. She also used the Timed Exercise Approach (TEA) format during the first few weeks. As explained earlier, this has a lot of advantages but none more imperative in this environment then allowing a FIT to focus on form rather than counting repetitions. Glancing at a stop watch while letting people work for an allotted amount of time allows for casual conversation among the group and the FIT to ensure they start to build a bond. Over the course of the next few weeks, that group started to build such a bond with one another they created their own W.O.W. t-shirts and would phone any absentee immediately after class to make sure they were okay. Having the group keep themselves accountable is a huge time saver and money maker for the FIT.

Carrie was charging $20/per person. The classes were limited to 10, and they were typically full. That is $200/hour in gross revenue. Even if you are giving a percentage to a facility or gym, running just a few of these per day you can make an absolute killing. Providing value to a specific population is the key. It can be done for any FIT if you use the tools and techniques we have discussed along the way here.

Burnout

You will be giving your all physically and emotionally day after day. Being a FIT is more taxing than people imagine. You'll have to avoid burnout, and I'll give you two strategies to do so, each from different timeline perspectives:

Short Term: Build in half hour breaks through-out your day. You will have to be "on" at all times and working too many classes or sessions in a row can reveal itself in negative ways. When you get a feel for how many hours you can work before there is a lull, write it down and the following week build in your half hour breaks. Recharging your batteries is ultimately the benefit of your client as they deserve your full attention, and for obvious safety concerns. On a weekly basis you should also leave a day with no training. This is for your friends, family, partner, and yourself. You will need the work/life balance to be a better FIT as it's all interconnected. If you are down in the dumps because you skipped out on seeing some friends in town to take on two additional training sessions, your clients will feel that negative energy. Being fully focused on your clients and career can only be done if your mind and body are allowed a weekly reboot. Recharge your batteries and make sure there aren't any programs running in the background so to speak.

Long Term: I was laid up after a double hernia surgery for three weeks. Not a single client left me, and in fact the majority of them dropped off homemade lunches and dinners by my house. If you've built a rapport through your good intentions and hard work, people will stick by you. Do not be concerned about taking vacations and trips with the fear of coming back to an empty schedule. Developing yourself through travel and leisure will ultimately make you a well-rounded FIT, and in turn attract more people to you. Your clients will like to know you have interests outside of work, and many times those interests will crossover, thereby causing a stronger bond.

6 - THE CEO OF YOU…BE RELENTLESS

"The amateur believes he must first overcome his fear; then he can do his work. The professional knows that fear can never be overcome."
— **Steven Pressfield, <u>The War of Art</u>**

Think honestly about the time you wake up in the morning, the effort you make the be a good employee, the seriousness you tackle tasks day after day, and then ponder this; Would you hire yourself? Maybe at your current position you wouldn't because it's just a "job" and not your ideal career. Moving forward however, do you think you'd be the ideal employee? Working 10% more hours in any industry has proven to give you a 40% pay increase. Understand that work to pay percentage is non-linear. You CAN out work people and earn a lot of money. This doesn't simply come from putting your nose to the grind. You need the perfect concoction of genuine reciprocity and internal drive to wake up each day understanding that you are the CEO of you.

Would you want your personal trainer to be half asleep or hung over from the night before? Clients are paying good money and choosing you as their expert FIT. We set examples for our client's health and habits. If you aren't eating, sleeping, and treating your body with the proper care, how can you expect them to, or for them to take your seriously?

We all have bad nights or even weeks, but in this gig remember that being "authentic" should be secondary to being a professional. If your surgeon had a fight the night before with his wife, and has been feeling a bit run down of late, do you want him to tell you, "Just to let you know, I am going to do this spinal fusion today, but I really wish I was home relaxing"? Your class or client are paying for your time, expertise, and fully-devoted attention and energy. You have to come to work prepared every day physically and psychologically. If you have an 8 a.m. appointment, you should be up at 6:55 a.m. mentally preparing yourself. You need to be just as attentive for your first client as your last. Not only is it a safety issue if you aren't on top of your game, but it's a disaster for long-term business success. Manic personality is not a trait that will help you as a FIT. You need to be cool, calm, and collected at all times.

Steven Pressfield, author of *War of Art*, talks about "resistance" and describes it as a, "…peripheral opponent…from within. It is self-generated and self-perpetuated." Seth Godwin, a public intellectual who has dozens of best sellers, refers to it as the "backward compass of the lizard brain", and that the vast majority of what we do comes from the subconscious, and only after the fact do we make up excuses or reasons why we decided to do so. Acknowledging that will help you come to grips that you did not inherit some internal struggle gene personalized to you, but rather that we all deal with this. There is no denying that it's tough to get out of bed at 5:00 a.m., and it's hard to find time to design workouts or prepare a choreographed class. Every job comes with its difficulties, but know that your shortcuts will hinder your long-term success as a FIT. Prepare yourself to shadow, make mistakes, and earn your way to the top through pushing past the resistance.

Routines will guide you into your success. Having a set routine that you don't skip out on trains your mind and body to set the habits permanence. Starting and keeping a routine is imperative. The phrase, "busy people get more done", or the "make the bed each morning" clichés puts you in the mindset of being task oriented in a timely manner. Set a routine, wake up at the same time, make sure you are fully alert and attentive, review your schedule for the day, bring materials that pertain to any particular special client/class, leave breaks to contact people if need be, check on all equipment and audio for your class/client, have food on hand to avoid "hangry" issues, and most importantly leave your psychological baggage at home.

The people who seem to not have the internal "resistance" struggles have simply learned through training to deal with obstacles like fear. It can also be done by you. By forcing yourself day-to-day to keep that upfront in consciousness will allow you to set a plan in place that allows your strategic decision-making to override your emotional drivers.

You are going to be put into situations that you don't feel comfortable with. Maybe it's teaching a particular demographic you've never worked with, or training someone for a sport you are unfamiliar with. These aren't things you should shy away from, but rather run toward. You'll make mistakes, but you'll learn to be a better FIT in the long term. These are just marbles being added to our career jar. There are no positive or negative marbles. The goal is to fill that mason jar, and every experience surrounding the profession helps us do just that. If you're prepared using the tools and techniques we discussed throughout the book, you'll be confident enough to handle these curveballs as you'll be comforted by already knowing you will swing and miss occasionally. A good FIT will always continue to learn and grow. I send thank you cards to my clients once a year, and in that card, I ask them to reevaluate their goals, as well as request they send me feedback on anything I can do better. It's important to be both hyper-confident in your ability and passion to help people, while also focusing on the reciprocity of the relationship. Your clients will become your friends, and you will learn as much from them as they do from you.

Like any other career, and potentially more so, there will be times (maybe weekly, or even daily) when you feel drained, and unmotivated. There will be instances when it feels like a job rather than the selfless educational lesson it is supposed to feel like. In each day of work, you will likely play the role of therapist, scientific researcher, nutritional advisor, news correspondent, restaurant critic, couples' counselor (oh yeah, get ready for the dirt), friend, and fitness guru. You will often be emotionally drained. You may feel as if you've worked twelve hours after only working six. However, it's all worth it if you've helped one of those six clients change their outlook on the day. I typically work 10-hour days because I love it; however, there are some days I cannot wait to go home and binge Amazon, Hulu, or Netflix (provided too many friends aren't signed into my account). What almost always happens during one of my last two sessions on a difficult day? A client who is truly in need comes in, and during our

"Update" phase spills the beans on their horrible week. "My husband is back in the hospital for the third time in two weeks. He has C-diff after having kidney stones, and his gall bladder removed. I've been looking forward to exercising and working out with you all week. What do you have planned for me today, Steve?" Go ahead, it's okay to cry. I swear to you not only has this exact story happened, but it happens to me regularly. During the "Update" phase I've had mothers confide in me about children recently lost in pregnancy, or their recent findings of their child's brain malformation needing surgery. I've had people tell me they are moving because of financial issues. I have had people recovering from near death car accidents work their way back to full health and credit our sessions as one of their main motivational factors. I've had hyper-successful millionaires tell me their therapists and medication don't hold a candle to one hour of exercise under my direction. These stories reinvigorate my passion to be a FIT, knowing that a person has chosen to spend an hour paying me with all that is going on in their lives. Life is tough, and we are all dealing with personal struggles. It's not simply part of your job, but rather your career's emphasis as a FIT to be ready, willing, and eager to not only listen and console your clients, but give them such a fantastic workout, coaching session, or class so for at least that one hour their burdens or stress are liberated.

That same instinctual selfless act that you would perform for a best friend without hesitation should be embedded in your fitness business endeavors. Ultimately, you'll only be successful in this business if your clients want to spend time with you. You have to create an environment that is positive, while simultaneously providing value as an expert in your field. If you focus on simply teaching people, learning from people, and booking sessions because you do not want to let down people who need exercise as their therapy (which they do), you **will** fill your schedule. You will build a unique friendship with your clients that allows the process of the financial transaction, yes giving you money, to almost never be discussed. People are intuitively attracted to others who have altruistic ideals and positive energy. They are willing to pay a small ransom if they are excited to both go into and leave your session knowing they will be in a better mood. The journey in getting to know your clients should be one in which you enjoy as much as helping them with whatever physical needs are necessary to address. In fact, helping them with their physical goals is sometimes only possible by first making sure they are in a healthy place psychologically. Regardless of the fitness medium, yoga, physical therapy, bootcamps, Pilates studio, speed training coach, you have to get to know your clients on some level or you will fail. Everyone I have worked with to this day I consider my friend. Clients will come to you because of your passion, willingness, knowledge, and relentless pursuit of doing the right thing session after session, day after day, like you would for your friends. I wish you all the luck in the universe. Go fill that mason jar!